BLOOD TYPE A DIET COOKBOOK FOR SENIOR

A Symphony of Wellness Through Tailored Diets, Gentle Exercises, and Stress

Herbert R. Anderson

Table of Contents

INTRODUCTION

Importance of Tailored Nutrition for Seniors

The importance of tailored nutrition for seniors lies at the intersection of advancing age, changing physiological needs, and the imperative to support overall health and well-being. As individuals age, their bodies undergo a multitude of changes, including alterations in metabolism, nutrient absorption, and the efficiency of various bodily functions. Tailored nutrition, specifically designed to meet the unique requirements of seniors, emerges as a crucial component in promoting optimal health and quality of life during the aging process.

Nutrient Absorption Efficiency:

- Seniors often experience a decline in the efficiency of nutrient absorption, which can lead to deficiencies in essential vitamins and minerals. Tailored nutrition takes into account these changes, focusing on nutrient-dense foods and appropriate supplements to address specific needs, such as calcium and vitamin D for bone health or B-vitamins for cognitive function.

Managing Chronic Health Conditions:

- Aging is frequently accompanied by an increased prevalence of chronic health conditions. Tailored nutrition strategies can play a pivotal role in managing and preventing these conditions. For instance, dietary adjustments can assist in controlling blood pressure, managing diabetes, and reducing the risk of cardiovascular diseases, all of which become more prevalent in the senior population.

Maintaining Healthy Weight:

Seniors often face challenges related to maintaining a healthy weight, either due to changes in metabolism or reduced physical activity. Tailored nutrition takes a comprehensive approach, ensuring that caloric intake aligns with energy expenditure while prioritizing nutrient density to support muscle mass and overall vitality.

Cognitive Function and Mental Health:

- Nutritional choices have a profound impact on cognitive function and mental health, aspects that gain significance as individuals age. Tailored nutrition emphasizes nutrients known to support brain health, such as omega-3 fatty acids, antioxidants, and certain vitamins, contributing to cognitive preservation and emotional well-being.

Digestive Health:

- Aging often brings about changes in digestive function, including a reduction in stomach acid production and potential alterations in gut microbiota. Tailored nutrition considers these factors, incorporating foods that are easy to digest, rich in fiber, and supportive of a healthy gut environment.

Promoting Immune Function:

- The immune system tends to undergo modifications with age, making seniors more susceptible to infections and illnesses. Tailored nutrition addresses immune health by including foods rich in antioxidants, vitamins, and minerals that contribute to the overall robustness of the immune system.

Enhancing Quality of Life:

- Ultimately, tailored nutrition aims to enhance the overall quality of life for seniors. By optimizing nutritional intake based on individual needs and health status, seniors are better equipped to maintain independence, energy levels, and vitality, fostering a sense of well-being as they navigate the aging process.

CHAPTER ONE

UNDERSTANDING BLOOD TYPE, A DIET

Characteristics of Blood Type A Individuals

Blood Type A individuals are characterized by specific traits and considerations that extend beyond their blood compatibility. While it's important to note that individual variations exist, here are some general characteristics associated with Blood Type A:

Adaptive Immune System:

- Blood Type A individuals often exhibit a balanced and adaptive immune response. They may have a slightly higher resistance to certain infections but may be more susceptible to others. This adaptability underscores the importance of personalized healthcare approaches.

Stress Sensitivity:

- Blood Type A individuals are commonly described as more sensitive to stressors, both physical and emotional. They may respond more acutely to stress, and managing stress becomes a crucial aspect of their overall well-being.

Personality Traits:

- While not universally applicable, some studies suggest that Blood Type A individuals may possess certain personality traits. They are often associated with characteristics such as conscientiousness, organization, and a tendency towards perfectionism.

Digestive Sensitivities:

- Blood Type A individuals may be more prone to digestive sensitivities, such as difficulty digesting certain proteins or a higher likelihood of gluten intolerance. Tailoring dietary choices to accommodate these sensitivities can contribute to better digestive health.

Dietary Recommendations:

- The Blood Type A diet typically recommends a plant-based eating pattern. This includes a focus on fresh, organic fruits and vegetables, legumes, and grains. It suggests minimizing the consumption of red meat and dairy products, aligning with a more vegetarian or pescatarian approach.

Cardiovascular Health Considerations:

- Some research suggests a potential association between Blood Type A and cardiovascular health. Blood Type A individuals may benefit from dietary habits that support heart health, such as including omega-3 fatty acids and maintaining a balanced intake of fats.

- **Fertility Considerations:** While ongoing research explores the connection between blood type and fertility, there may be specific considerations for Blood Type A individuals in reproductive health. Personalized fertility management plans may take blood type into account.

- **Blood Transfusion Compatibility:** In medical emergencies requiring blood transfusions, it's crucial to understand blood type compatibility. Blood Type A individuals can receive blood from donors with Blood Types A and O, highlighting the importance of accurate blood typing in healthcare settings.

Health Considerations for Blood Type A Seniors

Health considerations for Blood Type A seniors are of paramount importance, as the aging process brings about physiological changes that may require tailored approaches to support overall well-being. Understanding the unique characteristics of Blood Type, A individual allows for personalized healthcare strategies that address their specific needs.

Here are key health considerations for Blood Type A seniors:

Adapting to Changes in Immune Function:

- As seniors, Blood Type A individuals may experience changes in immune function. While they often possess an adaptive immune system, aging can impact immune responses. Strategies to support immune health, such as maintaining a nutrient-rich diet and staying active, become crucial in promoting resilience against infections.

Stress Management:

- Blood Type A seniors, known for their potential sensitivity to stress, should prioritize effective stress management techniques. Mindfulness practices, relaxation exercises, and engaging in activities that promote mental well-being can play a vital role in maintaining overall health.

Cognitive Health:

- Blood Type A individuals may have a predisposition towards conscientiousness, but cognitive health remains a consideration as they age. Incorporating foods rich in omega-3 fatty acids, antioxidants, and engaging in cognitive exercises can support brain health and potentially reduce the risk of age-related cognitive decline.

Digestive Sensitivities:

- Seniors often face changes in digestive function, and Blood Type A individuals may be more prone to digestive sensitivities. Adhering to the Blood Type A diet, which emphasizes plant-based foods and limits certain animal products, can contribute to digestive comfort and nutrient absorption.

Cardiovascular Health:

- Considering the potential association between Blood Type A and cardiovascular health, seniors should focus on heart-healthy habits. This includes maintaining a balanced diet, incorporating omega-3 fatty acids, managing blood pressure, and staying physically active to support cardiovascular well-being.

Bone Health:

- As seniors are susceptible to bone-related issues, Blood Type A individuals should ensure adequate intake of calcium and vitamin D, which are essential for bone health. Incorporating dairy alternatives, leafy greens, and exposure to sunlight can contribute to maintaining strong and healthy bones.

Joint Health:

- Aging may also bring about joint-related concerns. Blood Type A seniors can benefit from anti-inflammatory foods, such as those rich in omega-3 fatty acids, to support joint health. Engaging in low-impact exercises can also promote flexibility and reduce the risk of joint issues.

Regular Health Check-ups:

- Seniors, regardless of blood type, should prioritize regular health check-ups. Blood Type A individuals may have specific health considerations, and routine screenings can help detect and address potential issues early on. This includes monitoring cholesterol levels, blood pressure, and other indicators of overall health.

Social Engagement:

- Blood Type A seniors may thrive in environments that foster social connections. Social engagement has been linked to improved mental and emotional well-being. Encouraging participation in social activities, community events, or support groups can contribute to a fulfilling and health-promoting lifestyle.

Hydration and Nutrition:

- Proper hydration and adherence to the Blood Type A diet, which emphasizes plant-based foods, can contribute to maintaining optimal health. Seniors should focus on nutrient-dense foods that provide essential vitamins and minerals while staying adequately hydrated to support bodily functions.

CHAPTER TWO

BENEFITS OF BLOOD TYPE A DIET FOR SENIORS

Improved Digestion and Nutrient Absorption

Improved digestion and nutrient absorption are foundational elements of overall health, contributing to the body's ability to extract essential nutrients from the foods we consume. For individuals, including Blood Type A seniors, optimizing these processes becomes even more critical due to potential sensitivities and age-related changes. Let's professionally discourse the importance of improved digestion and nutrient absorption:

Digestive Efficiency in Blood Type A Seniors:

- Seniors, particularly those with Blood Type A, may experience changes in digestive function as part of the aging process. Enhancing digestive efficiency becomes crucial to ensure the proper breakdown of nutrients and absorption into the bloodstream. This is essential for maintaining optimal health and preventing nutritional deficiencies.

Impact of Blood Type on Digestive Preferences:

- Understanding the dietary preferences associated with Blood Type A is key to improving digestion. Blood Type A individuals often benefit from a plant-based diet, emphasizing fruits, vegetables, and legumes. Tailoring dietary choices to align with these preferences can contribute to smoother digestion and nutrient assimilation.

Reducing Digestive Discomfort:

- Blood Type A individuals may be prone to digestive sensitivities, such as gluten intolerance or difficulty digesting certain proteins. Modifying the diet to exclude or limit problematic foods can significantly reduce digestive discomfort, promoting a more comfortable and enjoyable eating experience for seniors.

Importance of Fiber for Seniors:

- Adequate fiber intake is crucial for seniors, and it aligns well with the Blood Type A diet recommendations. Fiber supports digestive health by promoting regular bowel movements and preventing constipation, which can become more prevalent in aging individuals. This, in turn, enhances the absorption of nutrients.

Supporting Gut Microbiota:

- The gut microbiota plays a pivotal role in digestion and nutrient absorption. Blood Type A seniors can benefit from incorporating probiotic-rich foods, such as yogurt or fermented vegetables, to support a healthy gut microbiome. A balanced and diverse microbiota contributes to efficient nutrient processing.

Hydration for Digestive Health:

- Proper hydration is fundamental for digestion and nutrient absorption. Blood Type A seniors should ensure an adequate intake of fluids, as dehydration can impede the digestive process. Drinking water throughout the day supports the breakdown of food and facilitates nutrient transport.

Optimizing Enzyme Production:

- Aging can affect the production of digestive enzymes, which are essential for breaking down nutrients into forms that the body can absorb. Blood Type A seniors may benefit from consuming enzyme-rich foods, such as pineapple and papaya, or considering enzyme supplements to enhance digestion.

Balancing Macronutrients:

- Blood Type A seniors can optimize digestion by balancing macronutrients in their diet. The Blood Type A diet emphasizes a balance of carbohydrates, proteins, and fats, tailored to individual needs. This balance promotes sustained energy levels and supports the efficient absorption of nutrients.

Mindful Eating Practices:

- Seniors, including Blood Type A individuals, can improve digestion through mindful eating practices. This involves paying attention to hunger and fullness cues, chewing food thoroughly, and avoiding distractions during meals. Such practices enhance the digestive process and nutrient assimilation.

Regular Monitoring and Adjustment:

- Blood Type A seniors should engage in regular monitoring of their digestive health. If concerns arise, adjustments to the diet or consulting with healthcare professionals can help address specific digestive issues promptly, ensuring optimal nutrient absorption.

Enhanced Immune Function

Enhanced immune function is a cornerstone of overall health and well-being, and its importance becomes particularly pronounced for individuals, including Blood Type A seniors, who may face age-related changes and potential health vulnerabilities. Professionally discussing the significance of enhanced immune function involves recognizing its role in preventing illness, promoting vitality, and addressing the unique considerations associated with Blood Type A individuals:

Foundations of Immune Health:

- A robust immune system forms the body's primary defense against pathogens and infections. For Blood

Type A seniors, maintaining optimal immune function is essential in safeguarding against illnesses and supporting longevity.

Adaptive Immune Response:

- Blood Type A individuals are often associated with an adaptable immune response. This adaptability can be leveraged to effectively respond to a variety of challenges, highlighting the importance of personalized healthcare approaches that recognize and utilize this characteristic.

Nutrition and Immune Health:

- Nutrition plays a pivotal role in immune function. Blood Type A seniors can enhance their immune health by aligning their dietary choices with the recommendations of the Blood Type A diet. Emphasizing immune-boosting nutrients such as vitamins C and E, zinc, and antioxidants becomes integral to supporting the immune system.

Anti-Inflammatory Lifestyle:

- Chronic inflammation can compromise immune function. Blood Type A seniors can benefit from adopting an anti-inflammatory lifestyle, including a diet rich in anti-inflammatory foods, regular physical activity, and stress management practices. These measures contribute to an environment that supports immune health.

Probiotics for Gut Health:

- The gut microbiota plays a significant role in immune regulation. Blood Type A seniors may consider incorporating probiotic-rich foods or supplements to support a healthy gut microbiome. A balanced and diverse microbiota enhances the immune system's ability to respond effectively to pathogens.

Adequate Sleep and Immune Function:

- Quality sleep is crucial for immune health. Blood Type A seniors should prioritize getting adequate and restful sleep, as it is during this time that the body undergoes essential repair and regeneration processes, contributing to a strengthened immune response.

Regular Physical Activity:

- Exercise has been linked to improved immune function. Blood Type A seniors can engage in regular, moderate-intensity physical activity, such as walking or yoga, to enhance circulation, promote overall health, and support immune function.

1. **Stress Management Strategies:** Chronic stress can suppress the immune system. Blood Type A individuals, known for potential stress sensitivity, should incorporate stress management strategies into their routine. Mindfulness, relaxation techniques, and engaging in

enjoyable activities contribute to a more resilient immune system.

2. **Hydration and Immune Support:** Proper hydration is fundamental for immune health. Blood Type A seniors should ensure they maintain adequate fluid intake, as hydration supports the transport of immune cells and the elimination of toxins from the body.

3. **Regular Health Check-ups:** Blood Type A seniors should undergo regular health check-ups to monitor their immune health and address any potential concerns promptly. Routine screenings, vaccinations, and discussions with healthcare professionals contribute to a proactive approach to immune support.

Managing Age-Related Health Issues

Managing age-related health issues is a multifaceted and dynamic process that requires a comprehensive and individualized approach, especially for individuals like Blood Type A seniors. As individuals age, they may encounter a range of health considerations, from chronic conditions to changes in physical and cognitive function. Professionally discussing the management of age-related health issues involves addressing these concerns with strategies that promote overall well-being and quality of life:

Holistic Health Assessment:

- The management of age-related health issues begins with a holistic health assessment. For Blood Type A seniors, understanding their unique characteristics, including potential sensitivities and predispositions, forms the foundation for personalized care plans. This assessment considers physical, mental, and emotional aspects of health.

Individualized Nutritional Approaches:

- Nutrition plays a pivotal role in managing age-related health issues. Blood Type A seniors can benefit from adhering to the dietary recommendations of the Blood Type A diet, which emphasizes a plant-based approach. Tailoring nutrition to support specific health needs, such as bone health or cardiovascular function, contributes to overall well-being.

1. **Regular Health Check-ups:** Routine health check-ups are essential for the early detection and management of age-related health issues. Blood Type A seniors should schedule regular appointments with healthcare professionals to monitor vital indicators, assess potential risk factors, and adjust healthcare strategies accordingly.

Cognitive Health Maintenance:

- Cognitive health becomes a significant consideration as individuals age. Blood Type A seniors can engage in activities that support cognitive function, such as mental exercises, social interactions, and a brain-healthy diet. Regular cognitive assessments can aid in identifying and addressing potential concerns early on.

Physical Activity and Mobility:

- Maintaining physical activity is crucial for managing age-related health issues, including joint health and cardiovascular function. Blood Type A seniors may benefit from exercises that align with their preferences and physical capabilities, such as walking, yoga, or swimming, to promote mobility and overall health.

Chronic Disease Management:

- Blood Type A seniors may be more prone to certain health conditions associated with aging. Managing chronic diseases, such as hypertension or arthritis, involves a collaborative approach between healthcare professionals and the individual. Medication management, lifestyle adjustments, and regular monitoring contribute to effective disease management.

Medication Review and Optimization:

- Seniors often take multiple medications, and regular review of medication regimens is critical. Blood Type A individuals should work closely with healthcare providers to optimize medication plans, address potential interactions, and ensure that medications align with their unique health considerations.

Mental and Emotional Well-being:

- Age-related health issues can impact mental and emotional well-being. Blood Type A seniors should prioritize activities that promote psychological health, such as engaging in hobbies, participating in social activities, and seeking support when needed. Managing stress and fostering resilience contribute to overall mental well-being.

Vision and Hearing Health:

- Blood Type A seniors should prioritize regular eye and ear examinations. Managing age-related changes in vision and hearing involves early detection of issues and addressing them with corrective measures, such as eyeglasses or hearing aids.

Social Connections and Support Systems:

- Maintaining strong social connections becomes increasingly important as individuals age. Blood Type A seniors can benefit from a supportive network of family, friends, and community. Social engagement contributes to mental well-being, provides emotional support, and enhances overall resilience.

CHAPTER THREE

BREAKFAST RECIPES

Quinoa Breakfast Bowl

Ingredients:

- 1 cup cooked quinoa
- 1/2 cup fresh berries (blueberries, raspberries)
- 1 tablespoon chia seeds
- 1 tablespoon almond butter
- 1 teaspoon honey

Prep Time: 5 minutes

Cooking Time: 10 minutes

Serving Time: Immediate

Nutritional Info: High in fiber, protein, and antioxidants

Instructions:

- In a bowl, combine cooked quinoa, fresh berries, chia seeds, and almond butter.
- Drizzle with honey for sweetness.
- Gently mix and serve.

Serving Methods:

1. Warm for a cozy breakfast.
2. Refrigerate overnight for a refreshing quinoa parfait.

Vegetable Omelette with Avocado

Ingredients:

- 2 eggs
- 1/4 cup diced bell peppers (various colors)
- 1/4 cup spinach, chopped
- 1/4 cup cherry tomatoes, halved
- 1/4 avocado, sliced

Prep Time: 10 minutes

Cooking Time: 8 minutes

Serving Time: Immediate

Nutritional Info: Rich in protein, vitamins, and healthy fats

Instructions:

- Whisk eggs and pour into a heated, oiled pan.
- Add bell peppers, spinach, and tomatoes to one half of the omelette.
- Fold the other half over the vegetables and cook until eggs are set.
- Serve with sliced avocado on top.

Serving Methods:

1. Roll the omelette for a breakfast wrap.
2. Pair with whole-grain toast for a heartier meal.

Green Smoothie Bowl

- ***Ingredients:***
- 1 cup kale, stems removed
- 1/2 banana
- 1/2 cup pineapple chunks
- 1/2 cup almond milk
- 1 tablespoon chia seeds

Prep Time: 5 minutes

Cooking Time: 0 minutes

Serving Time: Immediate

Nutritional Info: High in vitamins, minerals, and antioxidants

Instructions:

- Blend kale, banana, pineapple, and almond milk until smooth.
- Pour into a bowl and top with chia seeds.

Serving Methods:

1. Garnish with additional fruit for added freshness.
2. Sprinkle with granola or nuts for texture.

Sweet Potato and Spinach Hash

Ingredients:

- 1 cup sweet potatoes, diced
- 1 cup spinach, chopped
- 1/4 cup red onion, finely chopped

- 2 eggs

Prep Time: 10 minutes

Cooking Time: 15 minutes

Serving Time: Immediate

Nutritional Info: High in fiber, vitamins, and protein

Instructions:

- Sauté sweet potatoes and red onion in a pan until tender.
- Add spinach and cook until wilted.
- Create wells in the mixture and crack eggs into them.
- Cover and cook until eggs are done.

Serving Methods:

1. Top with avocado slices for added creaminess.
2. Serve over whole-grain toast for a complete meal.

Berry Almond Chia Pudding

Ingredients:

- 2 tablespoons chia seeds
- 1/2 cup almond milk
- 1/2 cup mixed berries (strawberries, blueberries)
- 1 tablespoon sliced almonds

Prep Time: 5 minutes

Cooking Time: 0 minutes (plus refrigeration time)

Serving Time: After refrigerating (about 4 hours)

Nutritional Info: High in omega-3s, antioxidants, and fiber

Instructions:

- Mix chia seeds and almond milk in a bowl. Let sit for a few minutes.
- Stir again and refrigerate until a pudding-like consistency forms.
- Layer with mixed berries and top with sliced almonds.

Serving Methods:

1. Blend into a smoothie for a quick breakfast drink.
2. Add a dollop of yogurt for extra creaminess.

Mushroom and Spinach Frittata

Ingredients:

- 4 eggs
- 1/2 cup mushrooms, sliced
- 1 cup spinach, chopped
- 1/4 cup feta cheese, crumbled

Prep Time: 15 minutes

Cooking Time: 20 minutes

Serving Time: Immediate

Nutritional Info: High in protein, iron, and vitamins

Instructions:

- Whisk eggs and pour into a greased baking dish.
- Sauté mushrooms and spinach until softened.
- Spread mushroom and spinach mixture over the eggs.
- Sprinkle feta cheese on top and bake until set.

Serving Methods:

1. Cut into squares for easy serving.
2. Pair with a side of sliced tomatoes for freshness.

7. Buckwheat Pancakes with Berries

Ingredients:

- 1/2 cup buckwheat flour
- 1/2 cup almond milk
- 1 egg
- 1/2 teaspoon baking powder
- 1/2 cup mixed berries (raspberries, blackberries)

Prep Time: 10 minutes

Cooking Time: 10 minutes

Serving Time: Immediate

Nutritional Info: Rich in fiber, antioxidants, and protein

Instructions:

- Mix buckwheat flour, almond milk, egg, and baking powder in a bowl.
- Heat a griddle and spoon batter onto it to form pancakes.
- Cook until bubbles appear, flip, and cook the other side.
- Serve with mixed berries on top.

Serving Methods:

1. Drizzle with a touch of honey for sweetness.
2. Top with a dollop of Greek yogurt for added creaminess.

Turmeric Smoothie with Mango

Ingredients:

- 1 cup mango chunks
- 1/2 teaspoon turmeric powder
- 1/2 cup Greek yogurt
- 1/2 cup coconut water
- 1 tablespoon flaxseeds

Prep Time: 5 minutes

Cooking Time: 0 minutes

Serving Time: Immediate

Nutritional Info: High in antioxidants, probiotics, and omega-3s

Instructions:

- Blend mango, turmeric, Greek yogurt, and coconut water until smooth.

- Pour into a glass and sprinkle flaxseeds on top.

Serving Methods:

1. Garnish with fresh mint leaves for added freshness.
2. Freeze into popsicle molds for a refreshing summer

Salmon and Avocado Breakfast Wrap

Ingredients:

- 1 whole-grain wrap
- 3 oz. smoked salmon
- 1/2 avocado, sliced
- 1 tablespoon Greek yogurt
- Fresh dill for garnish

Prep Time: 10 minutes

Cooking Time: 0 minutes

Serving Time: Immediate

Nutritional Info: Rich in omega-3s, protein, and healthy fats

Instructions:

- Lay the whole-grain wrap flat.
- Spread Greek yogurt over the wrap.
- Arrange smoked salmon and avocado slices.
- Garnish with fresh dill and fold into a wrap.

Serving Methods:

1. Cut into bite-sized pinwheels for a brunch platter.

2. Serve with a side of mixed greens for added freshness.

Blueberry Almond Flour Pancakes

Ingredients:

- 1 cup almond flour
- 2 eggs
- 1/2 cup almond milk
- 1/2 cup blueberries
- 1/2 teaspoon baking powder

Prep Time: 15 minutes

Cooking Time: 10 minutes

Serving Time: Immediate

Nutritional Info: High in protein, fiber, and antioxidants

Instructions:

- Whisk almond flour, eggs, almond milk, and baking powder in a bowl.
- Gently fold in blueberries.
- Spoon batter onto a griddle and cook until golden brown.

Serving Methods:

1. Top with a drizzle of maple syrup.
2. Serve with a dollop of coconut cream for a dairy-free option.

Spinach and Tomato Egg Muffins

Ingredients:

- 4 eggs
- 1 cup fresh spinach, chopped
- 1/2 cup cherry tomatoes, diced
- 1/4 cup feta cheese, crumbled
- Salt and pepper to taste

Prep Time: 10 minutes

Cooking Time: 20 minutes

Serving Time: Immediate

Nutritional Info: High in protein, vitamins, and minerals

Instructions:

- Preheat the oven to 350°F (175°C).
- In a bowl, whisk eggs and season with salt and pepper.
- Stir in chopped spinach, diced tomatoes, and crumbled feta.
- Pour the mixture into muffin cups and bake until set.

Serving Methods:

1. Serve with a side of sliced melon for a refreshing touch.
2. Sprinkle with fresh herbs like parsley or chives.

12. Coconut Chia Seed Pudding

Ingredients:

- 2 tablespoons chia seeds
- 1/2 cup coconut milk
- 1/4 cup pineapple chunks
- 1 tablespoon shredded coconut

Prep Time: 5 minutes

Cooking Time: 0 minutes (plus refrigeration time)

Serving Time: After refrigerating (about 4 hours)

Nutritional Info: Rich in omega-3s, fiber, and antioxidants

Instructions:

- Mix chia seeds and coconut milk in a bowl. Let sit for a few minutes.
- Stir again and refrigerate until a pudding-like consistency forms.
- Layer with pineapple chunks and shredded coconut.

Serving Methods:

1. Top with a dollop of Greek yogurt for added creaminess.
2. Garnish with mint leaves for a burst of freshness.

Turkey and Veggie Breakfast Skillet

Ingredients:

- 1/2 cup ground turkey
- 1/4 cup bell peppers, diced
- 1/4 cup zucchini, diced

- 2 eggs
- 1 tablespoon olive oil

Prep Time: 10 minutes

Cooking Time: 15 minutes

Serving Time: Immediate

Nutritional Info: High in protein, vitamins, and healthy fats

Instructions:

- In a skillet, heat olive oil and cook ground turkey until browned.
- Add diced bell peppers and zucchini.
- Create wells in the mixture, crack eggs into them, and cook until eggs are done.

Serving Methods:

1. Serve with a side of sliced avocado for added creaminess.
2. Sprinkle with chopped fresh herbs, such as cilantro or parsley.

Cinnamon Apple Quinoa Porridge

Ingredients:

- 1/2 cup cooked quinoa
- 1/2 apple, diced
- 1/4 teaspoon cinnamon

- 1 tablespoon almond butter
- 1 tablespoon maple syrup

Prep Time: 10 minutes

Cooking Time: 10 minutes

Serving Time: Immediate

Nutritional Info: High in fiber, antioxidants, and healthy fats

Instructions:

- In a saucepan, warm cooked quinoa with diced apples.
- Stir in cinnamon, almond butter, and maple syrup.
- Cook until apples are soft and the mixture is heated through.

Serving Methods:

1. Top with a sprinkle of chopped nuts for crunch.
2. Drizzle with coconut milk for added richness.

Avocado and Tomato Breakfast Toast

Ingredients:

- 2 slices whole-grain bread
- 1/2 avocado, mashed
- 1/2 cup cherry tomatoes, sliced
- Sprinkle of black sesame seeds

Prep Time: 5 minutes

Cooking Time: 5 minutes

Serving Time: Immediate

Nutritional Info: Rich in fiber, healthy fats, and vitamins

Instructions:

- Toast the whole-grain bread slices.
- Spread mashed avocado evenly on each slice.
- Arrange sliced cherry tomatoes on top.
- Sprinkle with black sesame seeds.

Serving Methods:

- Drizzle with balsamic glaze for added flavor.
- Serve with a side of mixed greens for extra freshness.

Mango and Almond Yogurt Parfait

Ingredients:

- 1/2 cup Greek yogurt
- 1/2 cup mango chunks
- 2 tablespoons granola
- 1 tablespoon sliced almonds

Prep Time: 5 minutes

Cooking Time: 0 minutes

Serving Time: Immediate

Nutritional Info: High in protein, fiber, and antioxidants

Instructions:

- In a glass, layer Greek yogurt, mango chunks, and granola.
- Repeat the layers until the glass is filled.
- Top with sliced almonds.

Serving Methods:

1. Drizzle with honey for added sweetness.
2. Freeze into popsicle molds for a refreshing summer treat.

Egg and Veggie Breakfast Burrito

Ingredients:

- 1 whole-grain tortilla
- 2 eggs, scrambled
- 1/4 cup black beans, cooked
- 1/4 cup salsa
- Fresh cilantro for garnish

Prep Time: 10 minutes

Cooking Time: 5 minutes

Serving Time: Immediate

Nutritional Info: High in protein, fiber, and vitamins

Instructions:

- Heat the whole-grain tortilla on a skillet.
- Fill with scrambled eggs, black beans, and salsa.
- Garnish with fresh cilantro before rolling into a burrito.

Serving Methods:

1. Top with a dollop of Greek yogurt for added creaminess.
2. Serve with a side of sliced melon for a refreshing touch.

Cherry Almond Smoothie Bowl

Ingredients:

- 1 cup cherries, pitted
- 1/2 banana
- 1/2 cup almond milk
- 1 tablespoon almond butter
- 2 tablespoons oats

Prep Time: 5 minutes

Cooking Time: 0 minutes

Serving Time: Immediate

Nutritional Info: High in antioxidants, fiber, and healthy fats

Instructions:

- Blend cherries, banana, almond milk, and almond butter until smooth.
- Pour into a bowl and sprinkle oats on top.

Serving Methods:

1. Add a swirl of coconut cream for extra richness.
2. Top with a handful of sliced almonds for crunch.

Peach and Walnut Overnight Oats

Ingredients:

- 1/2 cup rolled oats
- 1/2 cup almond milk
- 1 peach, sliced
- 1 tablespoon chopped walnuts
- 1 teaspoon honey

Prep Time: 5 minutes

Cooking Time: 0 minutes (plus refrigeration time)

Serving Time: After refrigerating (about 4 hours)

Nutritional Info: High in fiber, omega-3s, and vitamins

Instructions:

- Mix rolled oats and almond milk in a jar. Let sit for a few minutes.
- Layer with sliced peaches and chopped walnuts.
- Drizzle with honey before refrigerating.

Serving Methods:

1. Stir before serving for a creamy consistency.
2. Top with a scoop of yogurt for added richness.

Hazelnut and Raspberry Breakfast Muffins

Ingredients:

- 1 cup hazelnut flour
- 2 eggs
- 1/2 cup almond milk
- 1/2 cup fresh raspberries
- 1 tablespoon maple syrup

Prep Time: 15 minutes

Cooking Time: 20 minutes

Serving Time: Immediate

Nutritional Info: High in protein, antioxidants, and healthy fats

Instructions:

- Preheat the oven to 350°F (175°C) and line a muffin tin with liners.
- In a bowl, mix hazelnut flour, eggs, almond milk, and maple syrup.
- Gently fold in fresh raspberries.
- Spoon the batter into muffin cups and bake until set.

Serving Methods:

1. Drizzle with melted dark chocolate for a decadent touch.
2. Serve with a side of Greek yogurt for added creaminess.

CHAPTER FOUR

LUNCH RECIPES

Grilled Chicken Salad with Balsamic Vinaigrette

Ingredients:

- 4 oz. grilled chicken breast, sliced
- 2 cups mixed greens
- 1/2 cup cherry tomatoes, halved
- 1/4 cup cucumber, sliced
- 1/4 cup red bell pepper, diced
- 2 tablespoons feta cheese, crumbled

Prep Time: 15 minutes

Cooking Time: 10 minutes

Serving Time: Immediate

Nutritional Info: High in protein, vitamins, and antioxidants

Instructions:

- Season chicken breast with salt and pepper, grill until cooked.
- In a bowl, toss mixed greens, cherry tomatoes, cucumber, and red bell pepper.
- Top with sliced grilled chicken and crumbled feta.
- Drizzle with balsamic vinaigrette.

Serving Methods:

1. Serve in a wrap for a portable lunch option.

2. Garnish with toasted nuts for added crunch.

Quinoa and Vegetable Stir-Fry

Ingredients:

- 1 cup cooked quinoa
- 1/2 cup broccoli florets
- 1/2 cup snap peas
- 1/4 cup carrots, julienned
- 2 tablespoons soy sauce
- 1 tablespoon sesame oil

Prep Time: 15 minutes

Cooking Time: 10 minutes

Serving Time: Immediate

Nutritional Info: High in fiber, protein, and essential minerals

Instructions:

- In a wok, heat sesame oil and stir-fry broccoli, snap peas, and carrots.
- Add cooked quinoa and soy sauce, stir until well combined.
- Cook until vegetables are tender-crisp.

Serving Methods:

1. Stuff into bell peppers for a colorful presentation.

2. Top with sliced avocado for added creaminess.

Salmon and Avocado Wrap

Ingredients:

- 4 oz. baked salmon fillet, flaked
- 1 whole-grain wrap
- 1/4 cup Greek yogurt
- 1/2 avocado, sliced
- 1/4 cup mixed greens

Prep Time: 15 minutes

Cooking Time: 15 minutes

Serving Time: Immediate

Nutritional Info: Rich in omega-3s, protein, and healthy fats

Instructions:

- Bake salmon until cooked, then flake into chunks.
- Spread Greek yogurt on the whole-grain wrap.
- Arrange flaked salmon, avocado slices, and mixed greens.
- Roll into a wrap.

Serving Methods:

1. Cut into bite-sized pinwheels for a party platter.

Mushroom and Spinach Quiche

Ingredients:

- 1 whole-grain pie crust
- 4 eggs
- 1 cup mushrooms, sliced
- 1 cup spinach, chopped
- 1/2 cup feta cheese, crumbled
- 1/2 cup almond milk

Prep Time: 20 minutes

Cooking Time: 30 minutes

Serving Time: Immediate

Nutritional Info: High in protein, vitamins, and minerals

Instructions:

- Preheat the oven to 375°F (190°C).
- In a bowl, whisk eggs and almond milk.
- Line the pie crust with mushrooms, spinach, and feta.
- Pour the egg mixture over the ingredients.
- Bake until set and golden brown.

Serving Methods:

1. Serve with a side of mixed greens for freshness.
2. Cut into squares for easy serving.

Lentil and Vegetable Soup

Ingredients:

- 1 cup green lentils, cooked
- 1/2 cup carrots, diced
- 1/2 cup celery, chopped
- 1/2 cup onion, finely chopped
- 2 cloves garlic, minced
- 4 cups vegetable broth
- 1 teaspoon cumin
- 1 teaspoon turmeric

Prep Time: 15 minutes

Cooking Time: 25 minutes

Serving Time: Immediate

Nutritional Info: High in fiber, protein, and antioxidants

Instructions:

- In a pot, sauté onion and garlic until translucent.
- Add carrots, celery, cumin, and turmeric; cook for 5 minutes.
- Pour in vegetable broth and add cooked lentils.
- Simmer until vegetables are tender.

Serving Methods:

1. Garnish with fresh parsley for a burst of flavor.
2. Serve with a side of whole-grain crackers.

Greek Salad with Quinoa

Ingredients:

- 1 cup cooked quinoa
- 1/2 cup cucumber, diced
- 1/2 cup cherry tomatoes, halved
- 1/4 cup Kalamata olives, pitted
- 1/4 cup feta cheese, crumbled
- 2 tablespoons olive oil
- 1 tablespoon red wine vinegar

Prep Time: 15 minutes

Cooking Time: 15 minutes

Serving Time: Immediate

Nutritional Info: Rich in fiber, antioxidants, and healthy fats

Instructions:

- In a bowl, combine quinoa, cucumber, cherry tomatoes, olives, and feta.
- Drizzle with olive oil and red wine vinegar.
- Toss until well mixed.

Serving Methods:

1. Serve as a side dish with grilled chicken.
2. Stuff into hollowed-out bell peppers for a creative twist.

Sweet Potato and Chickpea Buddha Bowl

Ingredients:

- 1 cup roasted sweet potato cubes
- 1/2 cup cooked chickpeas
- 1/2 cup quinoa, cooked
- 1/4 cup red cabbage, shredded
- 2 tablespoons tahini dressing

Prep Time: 20 minutes

Cooking Time: 25 minutes

Serving Time: Immediate

Nutritional Info: High in fiber, protein, and vitamins

Instructions:

- Roast sweet potato cubes until golden brown.
- Arrange sweet potatoes, chickpeas, quinoa, and shredded red cabbage in a bowl.
- Drizzle with tahini dressing.

Serving Methods:

1. Top with sliced almonds for added crunch.
2. Serve in a large lettuce leaf for a low-carb option.

Turkey and Vegetable Stir-Fry

Ingredients:

- 1 cup lean ground turkey, cooked
- 1/2 cup broccoli florets
- 1/2 cup snow peas

- 1/4 cup bell peppers, sliced
- 2 tablespoons low-sodium soy sauce
- 1 tablespoon sesame oil

Prep Time: 15 minutes

Cooking Time: 10 minutes

Serving Time: Immediate

Nutritional Info: High in protein, fiber, and essential minerals

Instructions:

- In a wok, heat sesame oil and stir-fry ground turkey until browned.
- Add broccoli, snow peas, and bell peppers.
- Stir in low-sodium soy sauce until vegetables are tender.

Serving Methods:

1. Serve over cauliflower rice for a low-carb option.
2. Garnish with chopped green onions for added freshness.

Caprese Salad with Basil Pesto Dressing

Ingredients:

- 1 cup cherry tomatoes, halved
- 1/2 cup fresh mozzarella, diced
- 1/4 cup fresh basil leaves
- 2 tablespoons pine nuts
- 2 tablespoons basil pesto

Prep Time: 10 minutes

Cooking Time: 0 minutes

Serving Time: Immediate

Nutritional Info: Rich in vitamins, antioxidants, and healthy fats

Instructions:

- In a bowl, combine cherry tomatoes, fresh mozzarella, and basil leaves.
- In a dry skillet, toast pine nuts until golden brown.
- Add pine nuts to the salad and drizzle with basil pesto.

Serving Methods:

1. Serve on a bed of arugula for added peppery flavor.
2. Arrange on skewers for a delightful appetizer.

Cauliflower and Broccoli Soup

Ingredients:

- 1 cup cauliflower florets
- 1 cup broccoli florets
- 1/2 onion, chopped
- 2 cloves garlic, minced
- 4 cups vegetable broth
- 1/2 cup unsweetened almond milk
- Salt and pepper to taste

Prep Time: 15 minutes

Cooking Time: 25 minutes

Serving Time: Immediate

Nutritional Info: High in fiber, vitamins, and antioxidants

Instructions:

- In a pot, sauté onion and garlic until translucent.
- Add cauliflower, broccoli, and vegetable broth; simmer until vegetables are tender.
- Blend the mixture until smooth, then stir in almond milk.
- Season with salt and pepper.

Serving Methods:

1. Garnish with a dollop of Greek yogurt for added creaminess.
2. Serve with a sprinkle of chopped chives for extra flavor.

Eggplant and Lentil Stuffed Bell Peppers

Ingredients:

- 2 bell peppers, halved
- 1 cup cooked lentils
- 1 cup eggplant, diced
- 1/2 cup tomato sauce
- 1/4 cup red onion, finely chopped
- 2 tablespoons olive oil

Prep Time: 20 minutes

Cooking Time: 25 minutes

Serving Time: Immediate

Nutritional Info: High in fiber, protein, and antioxidants

Instructions:

- Preheat the oven to 375°F (190°C).
- In a skillet, sauté diced eggplant and red onion in olive oil until softened.
- Mix in cooked lentils and tomato sauce.
- Stuff bell peppers with the mixture and bake until peppers are tender.

Serving Methods:

1. Top with a sprinkle of nutritional yeast for a cheesy flavor.
2. Serve over a bed of quinoa for added protein.

Shrimp and Asparagus Stir-Fry

Ingredients:

- 8 oz. shrimp, peeled and deveined
- 1 cup asparagus, trimmed and cut into pieces
- 1/2 cup bell peppers, thinly sliced
- 2 tablespoons tamari sauce
- 1 tablespoon sesame oil

Prep Time: 15 minutes

Cooking Time: 10 minutes

Serving Time: Immediate

Nutritional Info: High in protein, vitamins, and essential minerals

Instructions:

- In a wok, heat sesame oil and stir-fry shrimp until pink.
- Add asparagus and bell peppers; cook until vegetables are tender.
- Stir in tamari sauce until well coated.

Serving Methods:

1. Serve over cauliflower rice for a low-carb option.
2. Garnish with sesame seeds for added crunch.

Chickpea and Cucumber Salad

Ingredients:

- 1 cup canned chickpeas, rinsed and drained
- 1/2 cucumber, diced
- 1/4 cup red onion, finely chopped
- 1/4 cup fresh parsley, chopped
- 2 tablespoons lemon juice
- 1 tablespoon olive oil

Prep Time: 10 minutes

Cooking Time: 0 minutes

Serving Time: Immediate

Nutritional Info: High in fiber, protein, and vitamins

Instructions:

- In a bowl, combine chickpeas, cucumber, red onion, and fresh parsley.
- Drizzle with lemon juice and olive oil.
- Toss until well mixed.

Serving Methods:

1. Serve on a bed of spinach for added greens.
2. Stuff into whole-grain pita pockets for a portable lunch.

Turkey and Quinoa Stuffed Peppers

Ingredients:

- 2 bell peppers, halved
- 1/2 cup cooked quinoa
- 1/2 cup lean ground turkey, cooked
- 1/4 cup black beans, cooked
- 1/4 cup salsa
- 1 teaspoon taco seasoning

Prep Time: 20 minutes

Cooking Time: 30 minutes

Serving Time: Immediate

Nutritional Info: High in protein, fiber, and essential minerals

Instructions:

- Preheat the oven to 375°F (190°C).
- In a bowl, mix cooked quinoa, ground turkey, black beans, salsa, and taco seasoning.
- Stuff bell peppers with the mixture and bake until peppers are tender.

Serving Methods:

1. Top with avocado slices for added creaminess.
2. Serve with a side of Greek yogurt for a cooling contrast.

Miso Glazed Tofu and Vegetable Skewers

Ingredients:

- 8 oz. firm tofu, cubed
- 1 cup bell peppers, cut into chunks
- 1 cup zucchini, sliced
- 1/4 cup miso paste
- 2 tablespoons rice vinegar
- 1 tablespoon maple syrup

Prep Time: 20 minutes

Cooking Time: 15 minutes

Serving Time: Immediate

Nutritional Info: High in protein, vitamins, and antioxidants

Instructions:

- In a bowl, whisk together miso paste, rice vinegar, and maple syrup.
- Thread tofu, bell peppers, and zucchini onto skewers.
- Brush with miso glaze and grill until vegetables are tender.

Serving Methods:

1. Serve over a bed of brown rice for a complete meal.
2. Garnish with sesame seeds and chopped green onions.

Egg Salad Lettuce Wraps

Ingredients:

- 4 hard-boiled eggs, chopped
- 1/4 cup celery, finely chopped
- 1/4 cup red onion, finely chopped
- 2 tablespoons Greek yogurt
- 1 tablespoon Dijon mustard
- Lettuce leaves for wrapping

Prep Time: 15 minutes

Cooking Time: 10 minutes

Serving Time: Immediate

Nutritional Info: High in protein, vitamins, and healthy fats

Instructions:

- In a bowl, combine chopped eggs, celery, red onion, Greek yogurt, and Dijon mustard.
- Mix until well combined.
- Spoon the egg salad into lettuce leaves and wrap.

Serving Methods:

1. Serve with a side of sliced tomatoes for freshness.
2. Top with avocado slices for added creaminess.

Sweet Potato and Black Bean Quesadillas

Ingredients:

- 2 whole-grain tortillas
- 1/2 cup mashed sweet potato
- 1/4 cup black beans, cooked
- 2 tablespoons salsa
- 1/4 cup shredded cheddar cheese

Prep Time: 15 minutes

Cooking Time: 10 minutes

Serving Time: Immediate

Nutritional Info: High in fiber, protein, and vitamins

Instructions:

- Spread mashed sweet potato on one side of each tortilla.
- Top with black beans, salsa, and shredded cheddar cheese.

- Fold in half and cook on a skillet until cheese is melted.

Serving Methods:

1. Cut into wedges and serve with a dollop of Greek yogurt.
2. Garnish with cilantro for added flavor.

Mediterranean Chickpea Salad

Ingredients:

- 1 cup canned chickpeas, rinsed and drained
- 1/2 cup cherry tomatoes, halved
- 1/2 cucumber, diced
- 1/4 cup Kalamata olives, pitted and sliced
- 2 tablespoons feta cheese, crumbled
- 2 tablespoons olive oil
- 1 tablespoon lemon juice

Prep Time: 15 minutes

Cooking Time: 0 minutes

Serving Time: Immediate

Nutritional Info: High in fiber, protein, and healthy fats

Instructions:

- In a bowl, combine chickpeas, cherry tomatoes, cucumber, olives, and feta.
- Drizzle with olive oil and lemon juice.
- Toss until well mixed.

Serving Methods:

1. Serve over a bed of arugula for a peppery kick.
2. Top with a sprinkle of dried oregano for a Mediterranean touch.

Vegetarian Lettuce Wraps with Tofu

Ingredients:

- 8 oz. extra-firm tofu, crumbled
- 1/2 cup water chestnuts, chopped
- 1/4 cup hoisin sauce
- 2 tablespoons soy sauce
- 1 tablespoon sesame oil
- Lettuce leaves for wrapping

Prep Time: 20 minutes

Cooking Time: 15 minutes

Serving Time: Immediate

Nutritional Info: High in protein, fiber, and essential minerals

Instructions:

- In a skillet, cook crumbled tofu until browned.
- Add water chestnuts, hoisin sauce, soy sauce, and sesame oil.
- Cook until well combined.
- Spoon the tofu mixture into lettuce leaves and wrap.

1. Top with sliced green onions for added freshness.
2. Serve with a side of pickled ginger for a zesty kick.

Cabbage and Turkey Sauté

Ingredients:

- 1 cup lean ground turkey, cooked
- 1 cup cabbage, shredded
- 1/2 cup carrots, julienned
- 1/4 cup soy sauce
- 1 tablespoon sesame oil

Prep Time: 15 minutes

Cooking Time: 15 minutes

Serving Time: Immediate

Nutritional Info: High in protein, vitamins, and essential minerals

Instructions:

- In a skillet, sauté ground turkey in sesame oil until browned.
- Add shredded cabbage and julienned carrots.
- Stir in soy sauce until vegetables are tender-crisp.

Serving Methods:

1. Serve over brown rice for a heartier meal.

2. Garnish with chopped cilantro for added flavor

CHAPTER FIVE

DINNER RECIPES

Baked Salmon with Lemon Dill Sauce

Ingredients:

- 6 oz. salmon fillet
- 1 tablespoon olive oil
- 1 tablespoon fresh dill, chopped
- 1 lemon, sliced
- Salt and pepper to taste

Prep Time: 10 minutes

Cooking Time: 20 minutes

Serving Time: Immediate

Nutritional Info: High in omega-3s, protein, and vitamins

Instructions:

- Preheat the oven to 375°F (190°C).
- Place the salmon on a baking sheet, drizzle with olive oil, and season with salt, pepper, and chopped dill.
- Arrange lemon slices on top of the salmon.
- Bake until the salmon is cooked through.

Serving Methods:

1. Serve over a bed of quinoa for added protein.
2. Pair with steamed asparagus for a balanced meal.

Stir-Fried Tofu and Vegetable Quinoa Bowl

Ingredients:

- 8 oz. extra-firm tofu, cubed
- 1 cup broccoli florets
- 1/2 cup bell peppers, sliced
- 1/4 cup snow peas
- 1 cup cooked quinoa
- 2 tablespoons tamari sauce

Prep Time: 15 minutes

Cooking Time: 15 minutes

Serving Time: Immediate

Nutritional Info: High in protein, fiber, and essential minerals

Instructions:

- In a wok, stir-fry tofu until golden brown.
- Add broccoli, bell peppers, and snow peas; cook until vegetables are tender-crisp.
- Stir in cooked quinoa and tamari sauce until well combined.

Serving Methods:

1. Top with a sprinkle of sesame seeds for added crunch.
2. Serve in lettuce cups for a low-carb option.

Turkey and Vegetable Stuffed Zucchini Boats

Ingredients:

- 2 medium zucchini
- 1/2 cup lean ground turkey, cooked
- 1/4 cup tomatoes, diced
- 1/4 cup red onion, finely chopped
- 2 cloves garlic, minced
- 2 tablespoons tomato sauce

Prep Time: 20 minutes

Cooking Time: 25 minutes

Serving Time: Immediate

Nutritional Info: High in protein, fiber, and vitamins

Instructions:

- Preheat the oven to 375°F (190°C).
- Cut zucchini in half lengthwise and scoop out the seeds.
- In a bowl, mix cooked ground turkey, tomatoes, red onion, garlic, and tomato sauce.
- Fill zucchini halves with the turkey mixture and bake until zucchini is tender.

Serving Methods:

1. Top with a dollop of Greek yogurt for added creaminess.
2. Serve over a bed of spinach for extra greens.

Quinoa and Vegetable Stuffed Bell Peppers

Ingredients:

- 2 bell peppers, halved
- 1 cup cooked quinoa
- 1/2 cup black beans, cooked
- 1/4 cup corn kernels
- 1/4 cup salsa
- 1 teaspoon cumin

Prep Time: 20 minutes

Cooking Time: 30 minutes

Serving Time: Immediate

Nutritional Info: High in protein, fiber, and essential minerals

Instructions:

- Preheat the oven to 375°F (190°C).
- In a bowl, mix cooked quinoa, black beans, corn, salsa, and cumin.
- Stuff bell peppers with the quinoa mixture and bake until peppers are tender.

Serving Methods:

1. Top with sliced avocado for added creaminess.
2. Serve with a side of Greek salad for a refreshing contrast.

Lemon Herb Chicken with Roasted Vegetables

Ingredients:

- 6 oz. chicken breast

- 1 tablespoon olive oil

- 1 teaspoon dried thyme

- 1 teaspoon dried rosemary

- 1 lemon, sliced

- Mixed vegetables (carrots, Brussels sprouts, sweet potatoes)

Prep Time: 15 minutes

Cooking Time: 30 minutes

Serving Time: Immediate

Nutritional Info: High in protein, vitamins, and antioxidants

Instructions:

- Preheat the oven to 400°F (200°C).

- Rub chicken with olive oil, thyme, and rosemary.

- Place chicken on a baking sheet surrounded by mixed vegetables.

- Arrange lemon slices over the chicken.

- Roast until chicken is cooked through and vegetables are tender.

Serving Methods:

1. Serve over a bed of quinoa for added protein.
2. Drizzle with a balsamic reduction for extra flavor.

Vegetarian Lentil Soup

Ingredients:

- 1 cup dried green lentils, rinsed
- 1/2 cup carrots, diced
- 1/2 cup celery, chopped
- 1/2 cup onion, finely chopped
- 2 cloves garlic, minced
- 4 cups vegetable broth
- 1 teaspoon cumin
- 1 teaspoon paprika

Prep Time: 15 minutes

Cooking Time: 30 minutes

Serving Time: Immediate

Nutritional Info: High in fiber, protein, and essential minerals

Instructions:

- In a pot, sauté onion and garlic until translucent.
- Add carrots, celery, cumin, and paprika; cook for 5 minutes.
- Pour in vegetable broth and add rinsed lentils.
- Simmer until lentils are tender.

Serving Methods:

1. Garnish with a dollop of Greek yogurt for added creaminess.

2. Serve with a side of whole-grain bread for a complete
   meal.

Shrimp and Broccoli Stir-Fry

Ingredients:

- 8 oz. shrimp, peeled and deveined
- 1 cup broccoli florets
- 1/2 cup snap peas
- 1/4 cup carrots, julienned
- 2 tablespoons low-sodium soy sauce
- 1 tablespoon sesame oil

Prep Time: 15 minutes

Cooking Time: 10 minutes

Serving Time: Immediate

Nutritional Info: High in protein, vitamins, and essential minerals

Instructions:

- In a wok, heat sesame oil and stir-fry shrimp until pink.
- Add broccoli, snap peas, and julienned carrots.
- Stir in low-sodium soy sauce until vegetables are tender.

Serving Methods:

1. Serve over cauliflower rice for a low-carb option.
2. Garnish with chopped green onions for added freshness.

Mushroom and Spinach Stuffed Chicken Breast

Ingredients:

- 6 oz. chicken breast
- 1/2 cup mushrooms, chopped
- 1 cup spinach, chopped
- 1/4 cup feta cheese, crumbled
- 1 tablespoon olive oil

Prep Time: 20 minutes

Cooking Time: 25 minutes

Serving Time: Immediate

Nutritional Info: High in protein, vitamins, and minerals

Instructions:

- Preheat the oven to 375°F (190°C).
- In a skillet, sauté mushrooms and spinach in olive oil until wilted.
- Butterfly the chicken breast and fill with the mushroom and spinach mixture.
- Sprinkle feta cheese on top.
- Bake until chicken is cooked through.

Serving Methods:

1. Serve with a side of roasted sweet potatoes for a balanced meal.
2. Drizzle with a balsamic glaze for extra flavor.

Cauliflower Rice Stir-Fry with Tofu

Ingredients:

- 8 oz. extra-firm tofu, cubed
- 1 cup cauliflower rice
- 1/2 cup bell peppers, sliced
- 1/4 cup snap peas
- 2 tablespoons tamari sauce
- 1 tablespoon sesame oil

Prep Time: 15 minutes

Cooking Time: 10 minutes

Serving Time: Immediate

Nutritional Info: High in protein, fiber, and essential minerals

Instructions:

- In a skillet, stir-fry tofu until golden brown.
- Add cauliflower rice, bell peppers, and snap peas; cook until vegetables are tender-crisp.
- Stir in tamari sauce until well combined.

Serving Methods:

1. Top with a sprinkle of sesame seeds for added crunch.
2. Serve in hollowed-out bell peppers for a creative presentation.

Lemon Garlic Shrimp with Zucchini Noodles

Ingredients:

- 8 oz. shrimp, peeled and deveined
- 2 zucchinis, spiralized into noodles
- 2 cloves garlic, minced
- 1 lemon, juiced and zested
- 2 tablespoons olive oil
- Fresh parsley for garnish

Prep Time: 15 minutes

Cooking Time: 10 minutes

Serving Time: Immediate

Nutritional Info: High in protein, vitamins, and healthy fats

Instructions:

- In a skillet, heat olive oil and sauté minced garlic until fragrant.
- Add shrimp and cook until pink.
- Stir in spiralized zucchini noodles, lemon juice, and zest.
- Cook until zucchini noodles are tender.

Serving Methods:

1. Garnish with fresh parsley for added flavor.
2. Serve with a side of roasted cherry tomatoes for sweetness.

Baked Cod with Herbed Quinoa

Ingredients:

- 6 oz. cod fillet
- 1 cup quinoa, cooked
- 1 tablespoon fresh parsley, chopped
- 1 tablespoon fresh dill, chopped
- 1 lemon, sliced
- Salt and pepper to taste

Prep Time: 15 minutes

Cooking Time: 20 minutes

Serving Time: Immediate

Nutritional Info: High in protein, fiber, and essential minerals

Instructions:

- Preheat the oven to 400°F (200°C).
- Place the cod fillet on a baking sheet, season with salt, pepper, and chopped herbs.
- Arrange lemon slices on top of the cod.
- Bake until the cod is cooked through and flaky.

Serving Methods:

1. Serve over herbed quinoa for a complete meal.
2. Pair with roasted Brussels sprouts for a nutritious side.

Chickpea and Spinach Curry

Ingredients:

- 1 cup canned chickpeas, rinsed and drained
- 1 cup spinach leaves
- 1/2 cup tomatoes, diced
- 1/4 cup red onion, finely chopped
- 2 tablespoons curry powder
- 1 tablespoon coconut oil

Prep Time: 15 minutes

Cooking Time: 20 minutes

Serving Time: Immediate

Nutritional Info: High in fiber, protein, and vitamins

Instructions:

- In a pan, sauté red onion in coconut oil until translucent.
- Add diced tomatoes, curry powder, chickpeas, and spinach.
- Cook until spinach wilts and chickpeas are heated through.

Serving Methods:

1. Serve over brown rice for a hearty meal.
2. Garnish with a dollop of coconut yogurt for creaminess.

Spaghetti Squash Primavera

Ingredients:

- 1 medium spaghetti squash

- 1/2 cup cherry tomatoes, halved
- 1/2 cup bell peppers, sliced
- 1/4 cup black olives, sliced
- 2 tablespoons olive oil
- Fresh basil for garnish

Prep Time: 15 minutes

Cooking Time: 30 minutes

Serving Time: Immediate

Nutritional Info: Low in carbs, high in vitamins, and antioxidants

Instructions:

- Preheat the oven to 375°F (190°C).
- Cut the spaghetti squash in half and remove seeds.
- Drizzle with olive oil, place face down on a baking sheet, and bake until tender.
- Use a fork to scrape the squash into "noodles."
- Toss with cherry tomatoes, bell peppers, and black olives.

Serving Methods:

1. Top with grilled chicken for added protein.
2. Garnish with fresh basil for a burst of flavor.

Turkey and Vegetable Skewers with Quinoa

Ingredients:

- 1 cup lean ground turkey, seasoned

- 1 cup bell peppers, cut into chunks
- 1 cup zucchini, sliced
- 1 cup cherry tomatoes
- 1 cup cooked quinoa
- 2 tablespoons balsamic glaze

Prep Time: 20 minutes

Cooking Time: 15 minutes

Serving Time: Immediate

Nutritional Info: High in protein, fiber, and essential minerals

Instructions:

- Preheat the grill or grill pan.
- Thread ground turkey, bell peppers, zucchini, and cherry tomatoes onto skewers.
- Grill until turkey is cooked and vegetables are tender.
- Serve over a bed of cooked quinoa and drizzle with balsamic glaze.

Serving Methods:

1. Serve with a side of mixed greens for freshness.
2. Pair with a whole-grain roll for a complete meal.

Lentil and Sweet Potato Casserole

Ingredients:

- 1 cup green lentils, cooked

- 1 large sweet potato, peeled and sliced

- 1/2 cup red onion, finely chopped

- 1/2 cup vegetable broth

- 2 tablespoons olive oil

- 1 teaspoon smoked paprika

Prep Time: 20 minutes

Cooking Time: 30 minutes

Serving Time: Immediate

Nutritional Info: High in fiber, protein, and vitamins

Instructions:

- Preheat the oven to 375°F (190°C).

- In a skillet, sauté red onion in olive oil until translucent.

- Layer sliced sweet potatoes in a baking dish.

- Mix cooked lentils, sautéed onions, vegetable broth, and smoked paprika.

- Pour lentil mixture over sweet potatoes and bake until sweet potatoes are tender.

Serving Methods:

1. Top with a sprinkle of nutritional yeast for a cheesy flavor.

2. Serve with a side of steamed broccoli for added greens.

Miso Glazed Eggplant with Quinoa

Ingredients:

- 1 large eggplant, sliced
- 1 cup quinoa, cooked
- 2 tablespoons miso paste
- 1 tablespoon rice vinegar
- 1 tablespoon maple syrup
- Sesame seeds for garnish

Prep Time: 15 minutes

Cooking Time: 20 minutes

Serving Time: Immediate

Nutritional Info: High in fiber, vitamins, and antioxidants

Instructions:

- Preheat the oven to 400°F (200°C).
- Lay eggplant slices on a baking sheet.
- In a bowl, whisk together miso paste, rice vinegar, and maple syrup.
- Brush the eggplant slices with the miso glaze and bake until tender.
- Serve over cooked quinoa and sprinkle with sesame seeds.

Serving Methods:

1. Top with sliced green onions for added freshness.
2. Pair with a side of pickled ginger for a zesty kick.

Salmon and Avocado Salad with Citrus Dressing

Ingredients:

- 6 oz. grilled salmon fillet, flaked
- 2 cups mixed greens
- 1/2 avocado, sliced
- 1/4 cup cherry tomatoes, halved
- 2 tablespoons orange juice
- 1 tablespoon olive oil

Prep Time: 15 minutes

Cooking Time: 10 minutes

Serving Time: Immediate

Nutritional Info: High in omega-3s, vitamins, and healthy fats

Instructions:

- Grill the salmon until cooked through and flake into pieces.
- In a bowl, toss mixed greens, avocado slices, and cherry tomatoes.
- Whisk together orange juice and olive oil to create the dressing.
- Drizzle the dressing over the salad and top with grilled salmon.

Serving Methods:

1. Sprinkle with crushed nuts for added texture.
2. Serve with a side of quinoa for a more substantial meal.

Stuffed Portobello Mushrooms with Spinach and Feta

Ingredients:

- 2 large Portobello mushrooms, stems removed
- 1 cup spinach, sautéed
- 1/4 cup feta cheese, crumbled
- 2 tablespoons balsamic glaze
- Fresh basil for garnish

Prep Time: 15 minutes

Cooking Time: 20 minutes

Serving Time: Immediate

Nutritional Info: High in fiber, vitamins, and minerals

Instructions:

- Preheat the oven to 375°F (190°C).
- Place Portobello mushrooms on a baking sheet.
- Fill each mushroom with sautéed spinach and crumbled feta.
- Bake until mushrooms are tender.
- Drizzle with balsamic glaze and garnish with fresh basil.

Serving Methods:

1. Serve over a bed of arugula for added peppery flavor.
2. Pair with a side of quinoa for extra protein.

Chicken and Broccoli Quinoa Bowl

Ingredients:

- 6 oz. chicken breast, grilled and sliced
- 1 cup broccoli florets, steamed
- 1 cup cooked quinoa
- 2 tablespoons tahini dressing
- Sesame seeds for garnish

Prep Time: 15 minutes

Cooking Time: 20 minutes

Serving Time: Immediate

Nutritional Info: High in protein, fiber, and essential minerals

Instructions:

- Grill the chicken until cooked through and slice into strips.
- Steam broccoli florets until tender-crisp.
- In a bowl, combine cooked quinoa, grilled chicken, and steamed broccoli.
- Drizzle with tahini dressing and sprinkle with sesame seeds.

Serving Methods:

1. Serve in lettuce cups for a low-carb option.
2. Garnish with chopped green onions for added freshness.

Vegetable and Tofu Stir-Fry with Brown Rice

Ingredients:

- 8 oz. firm tofu, cubed
- 1 cup broccoli florets
- 1/2 cup carrots, julienned
- 1/2 cup snap peas
- 1 cup brown rice, cooked
- 2 tablespoons low-sodium soy sauce

Prep Time: 20 minutes

Cooking Time: 15 minutes

Serving Time: Immediate

Nutritional Info: High in protein, fiber, and essential minerals

Instructions:

- In a wok, stir-fry tofu until golden brown.
- Add broccoli, carrots, and snap peas; cook until vegetables are tender-crisp.
- Stir in low-sodium soy sauce until well combined.
- Serve over cooked brown rice.

Serving Methods:

1. Top with sliced green onions for added freshness.
2. Garnish with sesame seeds for extra crunch.

CHAPTER SIX

SNACKS RECIPES

Greek Yogurt Parfait

Ingredients:

- 1 cup Greek yogurt
- 1/2 cup mixed berries (blueberries, strawberries)
- 1 tablespoon honey
- 2 tablespoons granola

Prep Time: 5 minutes

Cooking Time: 0 minutes

Serving Time: Immediate

Nutritional Info: High in protein, probiotics, and antioxidants

Instructions:

- In a glass or bowl, layer Greek yogurt, mixed berries, and granola.
- Drizzle honey over the top.
- Repeat layers and serve.

Serving Methods:

1. Garnish with mint leaves for a fresh touch.
2. Serve in small jars for a portable snack.

Almond Butter and Banana Rice Cakes

Ingredients:

- 2 rice cakes
- 2 tablespoons almond butter
- 1 banana, sliced
- Chia seeds for garnish

Prep Time: 5 minutes

Cooking Time: 0 minutes

Serving Time: Immediate

Nutritional Info: High in protein, healthy fats, and potassium

Instructions:

- Spread almond butter evenly on rice cakes.
- Top with banana slices.
- Sprinkle chia seeds on top.

Serving Methods:

1. Drizzle with a touch of honey for sweetness.
2. Serve with a side of unsweetened almond milk.

Roasted Chickpeas with Herbs

Ingredients:

- 1 can chickpeas, drained and rinsed
- 1 tablespoon olive oil
- 1 teaspoon dried rosemary
- 1 teaspoon garlic powder

- Salt and pepper to taste

Prep Time: 5 minutes

Cooking Time: 25 minutes

Serving Time: Immediate

Nutritional Info: High in protein, fiber, and vitamins

Instructions:

- Preheat the oven to 400°F (200°C).
- Toss chickpeas with olive oil, rosemary, garlic powder, salt, and pepper.
- Roast on a baking sheet until crispy.

Serving Methods:

1. Sprinkle nutritional yeast for a cheesy flavor.
2. Serve in small bowls for portion control.

Cucumber and Hummus Bites

Ingredients:

- 1 cucumber, sliced
- 1/2 cup hummus
- Cherry tomatoes for topping
- Fresh dill for garnish

Prep Time: 10 minutes

Cooking Time: 0 minutes

Serving Time: Immediate

Nutritional Info: High in fiber, healthy fats, and vitamins

Instructions:

- Spread hummus on cucumber slices.
- Top with cherry tomatoes.
- Garnish with fresh dill.

Serving Methods:

1. Drizzle with extra virgin olive oil for richness.
2. Serve on a platter for a visually appealing snack.

Trail Mix with Nuts and Dried Fruit

Ingredients:

- 1/4 cup almonds
- 1/4 cup walnuts
- 2 tablespoons pumpkin seeds
- 2 tablespoons dried cranberries
- 2 tablespoons dark chocolate chips

Prep Time: 5 minutes

Cooking Time: 0 minutes

Serving Time: Immediate

Nutritional Info: High in healthy fats, antioxidants, and minerals

Instructions:

- Mix almonds, walnuts, pumpkin seeds, dried cranberries, and dark chocolate chips in a bowl.
- Toss until well combined.

Serving Methods:

1. Portion into small snack-sized bags for on-the-go.
2. Sprinkle over Greek yogurt for a crunchy topping.

Apple Slices with Almond Butter

Ingredients:

- 1 apple, sliced
- 2 tablespoons almond butter
- Cinnamon for sprinkling

Prep Time: 5 minutes

Cooking Time: 0 minutes

Serving Time: Immediate

Nutritional Info: High in fiber, healthy fats, and antioxidants

Instructions:

- Spread almond butter on apple slices.
- Sprinkle with cinnamon.

Serving Methods:

1. Top with chia seeds for added texture.
2. Serve with a side of herbal tea for a cozy snack.

Mango Salsa with Jicama Sticks

Ingredients:

- 1 mango, diced
- 1/2 red bell pepper, finely chopped
- 1/4 red onion, finely chopped
- 1 tablespoon cilantro, chopped
- Jicama sticks for dipping

Prep Time: 10 minutes

Cooking Time: 0 minutes

Serving Time: Immediate

Nutritional Info: High in vitamins, fiber, and antioxidants

Instructions:

- In a bowl, mix diced mango, red bell pepper, red onion, and cilantro.
- Stir until well combined.

Serving Methods:

1. Squeeze fresh lime juice over the salsa for brightness.
2. Serve with jicama sticks for a refreshing crunch.

Chia Pudding with Berries

Ingredients:

- 2 tablespoons chia seeds

- 1/2 cup almond milk
- 1/2 teaspoon vanilla extract
- Mixed berries for topping

Prep Time: 5 minutes

Cooking Time: 0 minutes

Serving Time: 2 hours (for chia pudding to set)

Nutritional Info: High in fiber, omega-3s, and antioxidants

Instructions:

- In a jar, mix chia seeds, almond milk, and vanilla extract.
- Stir well, cover, and refrigerate for at least 2 hours or overnight.
- Top with mixed berries before serving.

Serving Methods:

1. Drizzle with honey for sweetness.
2. Layer with granola for added crunch.

Sweet Potato Toast with Avocado

Ingredients:

- 1 sweet potato, sliced and roasted
- 1/2 avocado, mashed
- Red pepper flakes for sprinkling
- Sesame seeds for garnish

Prep Time: 15 minutes

Cooking Time: 15 minutes

Serving Time: Immediate

Nutritional Info: High in fiber, healthy fats, and vitamins

Instructions:

- Slice sweet potato into thin rounds and roast until tender.
- Spread mashed avocado on sweet potato rounds.
- Sprinkle with red pepper flakes and sesame seeds.

Serving Methods:

1. Top with a poached egg for added protein.
2. Serve on a wooden board for an appetizing presentation.

Caprese Skewers

Ingredients:

- Cherry tomatoes
- Fresh mozzarella balls
- Basil leaves
- Balsamic glaze for drizzling

Prep Time: 10 minutes

Cooking Time: 0 minutes

Serving Time: Immediate

Nutritional Info: High in protein, calcium, and vitamins

Instructions:

- Thread a cherry tomato, fresh mozzarella ball, and basil leaf onto small skewers.
- Arrange on a serving platter.
- Drizzle with balsamic glaze before serving.

Serving Methods:

1. Sprinkle with sea salt for enhanced flavor.
2. Serve alongside whole-grain crackers for a more substantial snack.

Edamame Guacamole

Ingredients:

- 1 cup edamame, shelled and cooked
- 1 avocado, mashed
- 1/4 cup red onion, finely chopped
- 1 clove garlic, minced
- Lime juice for acidity

Prep Time: 10 minutes

Cooking Time: 5 minutes

Serving Time: Immediate

Nutritional Info: High in protein, healthy fats, and vitamins

Instructions:

- In a food processor, blend edamame until finely chopped.

- Combine mashed avocado, chopped red onion, minced garlic, and lime juice.
- Mix until well combined.

Serving Methods:

1. Sprinkle with pumpkin seeds for added crunch.
2. Serve with sliced cucumber for a low-carb option.

Quinoa Stuffed Bell Peppers

Ingredients:

- Mini bell peppers, halved
- 1 cup cooked quinoa
- 1/2 cup black beans, rinsed
- 1/4 cup cherry tomatoes, diced
- 1/4 cup cilantro, chopped

Prep Time: 15 minutes

Cooking Time: 0 minutes

Serving Time: Immediate

Nutritional Info: High in fiber, protein, and essential minerals

Instructions:

- In a bowl, mix cooked quinoa, black beans, diced cherry tomatoes, and chopped cilantro.
- Stuff mini bell peppers with the quinoa mixture.

Serving Methods:

1. Top with a dollop of Greek yogurt for creaminess.

2. Sprinkle with nutritional yeast for a cheesy flavor.

Spiced Almonds

Ingredients:

- 1 cup raw almonds
- 1 tablespoon olive oil
- 1 teaspoon smoked paprika
- 1/2 teaspoon cayenne pepper
- Sea salt to taste

Prep Time: 5 minutes

Cooking Time: 10 minutes

Serving Time: Immediate

Nutritional Info: High in healthy fats, protein, and antioxidants

Instructions:

- Preheat the oven to 350°F (175°C).
- In a bowl, toss almonds with olive oil, smoked paprika, cayenne pepper, and sea salt.
- Spread the almonds on a baking sheet and roast until fragrant.

Serving Methods:

1. Mix with dried cranberries for a sweet and spicy trail mix.

2. Serve in small jars for a convenient snack.

Blueberry Chia Seed Pudding

Ingredients:

- 1/4 cup chia seeds
- 1 cup almond milk
- 1/2 teaspoon vanilla extract
- 1/2 cup blueberries

Prep Time: 5 minutes

Cooking Time: 0 minutes

Serving Time: 2 hours (for chia pudding to set)

Nutritional Info: High in fiber, omega-3s, and antioxidants

Instructions:

- In a jar, mix chia seeds, almond milk, and vanilla extract.
- Stir well, cover, and refrigerate for at least 2 hours or overnight.
- Top with fresh blueberries before serving.

Serving Methods:

1. Drizzle with a touch of honey for sweetness.
2. Layer with sliced strawberries for variety.

Avocado and Tomato Salsa

Ingredients:

- 1 avocado, diced

- 1 cup cherry tomatoes, halved
- 1/4 cup red onion, finely chopped
- 2 tablespoons fresh cilantro, chopped
- Lime juice for acidity

Prep Time: 10 minutes

Cooking Time: 0 minutes

Serving Time: Immediate

Nutritional Info: High in healthy fats, vitamins, and antioxidants

Instructions:

- In a bowl, combine diced avocado, cherry tomatoes, chopped red onion, and cilantro.
- Drizzle with lime juice and toss gently.

Serving Methods:

1. Serve with whole-grain pita chips for dipping.
2. Spoon over rice cakes for a light and crunchy snack.

Sesame Ginger Snap Peas

Ingredients:

- 1 cup snap peas, ends trimmed
- 1 tablespoon sesame oil
- 1 teaspoon grated ginger
- Sesame seeds for garnish

Prep Time: 5 minutes

Cooking Time: 5 minutes

Serving Time: Immediate

Nutritional Info: High in fiber, vitamins, and essential minerals

Instructions:

- In a pan, heat sesame oil and sauté snap peas until tender-crisp.
- Add grated ginger and toss until evenly coated.
- Sprinkle with sesame seeds before serving.

Serving Methods:

Serve chilled for a refreshing snack.

Pair with a cup of green tea for a delightful combination.

Cottage Cheese and Pineapple Cups

Ingredients:

- 1 cup low-fat cottage cheese
- 1/2 cup fresh pineapple, diced
- 1 tablespoon shredded coconut
- Mint leaves for garnish

Prep Time: 5 minutes

Cooking Time: 0 minutes

Serving Time: Immediate

Nutritional Info: High in protein, vitamins, and healthy fats

Instructions:

- In a bowl, mix cottage cheese with diced pineapple.
- Spoon the mixture into small cups.
- Sprinkle shredded coconut on top and garnish with mint leaves.

Serving Methods:

1. Drizzle with honey for a touch of sweetness.
2. Serve with whole-grain crackers for added texture.

Whole Grain Toast with Smoked Salmon

Ingredients:

- 2 slices whole grain bread, toasted
- 2 oz. smoked salmon
- 1 tablespoon cream cheese
- Fresh dill for garnish

Prep Time: 5 minutes

Cooking Time: 0 minutes

Serving Time: Immediate

Nutritional Info: High in omega-3s, fiber, and protein

Instructions:

- Spread cream cheese on toasted whole grain bread.
- Top with smoked salmon.
- Garnish with fresh dill.

Serving Methods:

1. Add capers for an extra burst of flavor.
2. Serve on a wooden board for an elegant presentation.

Homemade Veggie Chips

Ingredients:

- 1 sweet potato, thinly sliced
- 1 zucchini, thinly sliced
- 1 beet, thinly sliced
- 2 tablespoons olive oil
- Sea salt for seasoning

Prep Time: 15 minutes

Cooking Time: 20 minutes

Serving Time: Immediate

Nutritional Info: High in fiber, vitamins, and antioxidants

Instructions:

- Preheat the oven to 375°F (190°C).
- Toss sweet potato, zucchini, and beet slices with olive oil.
- Spread on a baking sheet and bake until crispy.
- Season with sea salt.

Serving Methods:

1. Pair with a homemade yogurt dip for added creaminess.
2. Serve in colorful bowls for a visually appealing snack.

Pomegranate and Feta Bites

Ingredients:

- 1 cup pomegranate arils
- 1/2 cup feta cheese, crumbled
- 1 tablespoon balsamic glaze
- Fresh mint for garnish

Prep Time: 10 minutes

Cooking Time: 0 minutes

Serving Time: Immediate

Nutritional Info: High in antioxidants, calcium, and vitamins

Instructions:

- In a bowl, combine pomegranate arils and crumbled feta.
- Drizzle with balsamic glaze and toss gently.
- Garnish with fresh mint.

Serving Methods:

1. Serve on skewers for a festive presentation.
2. Sprinkle with crushed pistachios for added crunch.

CHAPTER SEVEN

DESSERTS RECIPES

Chia Seed Pudding with Mixed Berries

Ingredients:

- 2 tablespoons chia seeds
- 1 cup almond milk
- 1/2 teaspoon vanilla extract
- Mixed berries for topping

Prep Time: 5 minutes

Cooking Time: 0 minutes

Serving Time: 2 hours (for chia pudding to set)

Nutritional Info: High in fiber, omega-3s, and antioxidants

Instructions:

- In a jar, mix chia seeds, almond milk, and vanilla extract.
- Stir well, cover, and refrigerate for at least 2 hours or overnight.
- Top with a variety of mixed berries before serving.

Serving Methods:

1. Layer with granola for added crunch.
2. Garnish with a dollop of Greek yogurt for creaminess.

Baked Apple with Cinnamon and Almonds

Ingredients:

- 1 apple, cored and sliced
- 1 teaspoon cinnamon
- 1 tablespoon slivered almonds
- 1 teaspoon honey

Prep Time: 10 minutes

Cooking Time: 20 minutes

Serving Time: Immediate

Nutritional Info: High in fiber, antioxidants, and healthy fats

Instructions:

Preheat the oven to 375°F (190°C).

Place apple slices on a baking sheet, sprinkle with cinnamon, and top with slivered almonds.

Bake until apples are tender.

Drizzle with honey before serving.

Serving Methods:

1. Serve with a scoop of vanilla Greek yogurt for added richness.
2. Top with a sprinkle of chia seeds for an extra nutritional boost.

Avocado Chocolate Mousse

Ingredients:

- 2 ripe avocados
- 1/4 cup unsweetened cocoa powder
- 1/4 cup maple syrup
- 1 teaspoon vanilla extract

Prep Time: 10 minutes

Cooking Time: 0 minutes

Serving Time: Immediate

Nutritional Info: High in healthy fats, antioxidants, and vitamins

Instructions:

- In a blender, combine ripe avocados, cocoa powder, maple syrup, and vanilla extract.
- Blend until smooth and creamy.
- Chill in the refrigerator for at least 30 minutes before serving.

Serving Methods:

1. Top with fresh raspberries for a burst of flavor.
2. Serve in small ramekins for portion control.

Coconut and Berry Parfait

Ingredients:

- 1 cup coconut yogurt
- 1/2 cup mixed berries (strawberries, blueberries)
- 2 tablespoons shredded coconut
- 1 tablespoon honey

Prep Time: 5 minutes

Cooking Time: 0 minutes

Serving Time: Immediate

Nutritional Info: High in probiotics, antioxidants, and healthy fats

Instructions:

- In a glass or bowl, layer coconut yogurt and mixed berries.
- Sprinkle shredded coconut on top.
- Drizzle with honey before serving.

Serving Methods:

1. Top with a handful of granola for added texture.
2. Garnish with mint leaves for freshness.

Banana and Walnut Bread

Ingredients:

- 2 ripe bananas, mashed
- 1 cup almond flour
- 1/4 cup coconut flour

- 1/2 cup walnuts, chopped
- 1 teaspoon baking powder
- 1/2 teaspoon cinnamon

Prep Time: 10 minutes

Cooking Time: 30 minutes

Serving Time: Immediate

Nutritional Info: High in fiber, healthy fats, and potassium

Instructions:

- Preheat the oven to 350°F (175°C).
- In a bowl, mix mashed bananas, almond flour, coconut flour, chopped walnuts, baking powder, and cinnamon.
- Pour into a greased loaf pan and bake until a toothpick comes out clean.

Serving Methods:

1. Slice and serve with a dollop of almond butter.
2. Top with a scoop of dairy-free ice cream for a treat.

Mango Sorbet with Mint

Ingredients:

- 2 cups frozen mango chunks
- 1/4 cup coconut water
- Fresh mint leaves for garnish

Prep Time: 5 minutes

Cooking Time: 0 minutes

Serving Time: Immediate

Nutritional Info: High in vitamins, antioxidants, and hydration

Instructions:

- In a blender, blend frozen mango chunks and coconut water until smooth.
- Scoop into bowls or glasses.
- Garnish with fresh mint leaves before serving.

Serving Methods:

1. Top with a sprinkle of chia seeds for added crunch.
2. Serve with a side of sliced kiwi for a tropical twist.

Berry and Almond Tart

Ingredients:

- 1 cup almond flour
- 1/4 cup coconut oil, melted
- 1 tablespoon maple syrup
- 1 cup mixed berries (raspberries, blackberries)
- 1 tablespoon sliced almonds

Prep Time: 15 minutes

Cooking Time: 15 minutes

Serving Time: Immediate

Nutritional Info: High in fiber, healthy fats, and antioxidants

Instructions:

- Preheat the oven to 350°F (175°C).
- In a bowl, mix almond flour, melted coconut oil, and maple syrup to form a crust.
- Press the mixture into a tart pan and bake until golden.
- Once cooled, top with mixed berries and sliced almonds.

Serving Methods:

1. Drizzle with a balsamic reduction for a gourmet touch.
2. Serve with a dollop of coconut whipped cream.

Matcha Green Tea Popsicles

Ingredients:

- 1 cup coconut milk
- 1 teaspoon matcha green tea powder
- 2 tablespoons honey
- Sliced kiwi for layering

Prep Time: 10 minutes

Freezing Time: 4 hours

Serving Time: Immediate

Nutritional Info: High in antioxidants, healthy fats, and vitamins

Instructions:

- In a bowl, whisk together coconut milk, matcha powder, and honey until well combined.
- Pour a layer of the mixture into popsicle molds.
- Add a layer of sliced kiwi and repeat until molds are filled.
- Insert popsicle sticks and freeze for at least 4 hours.

Serving Methods:

1. Dip in melted dark chocolate for an indulgent treat.
2. Serve with a sprinkle of crushed pistachios for added texture.

Pumpkin Spice Baked Apples

Ingredients:

- 2 apples, cored and halved
- 1/4 cup pumpkin puree
- 1 tablespoon maple syrup
- 1/2 teaspoon pumpkin spice

Prep Time: 10 minutes

Cooking Time: 25 minutes

Serving Time: Immediate

Nutritional Info: High in fiber, vitamins, and antioxidants

Instructions:

- Preheat the oven to 375°F (190°C).

- In a bowl, mix pumpkin puree, maple syrup, and pumpkin spice.
- Hollow out apples and fill with the pumpkin mixture.
- Bake until apples are tender.

Serving Methods:

1. Top with a sprinkle of chopped pecans for crunch.
2. Serve with a scoop of non-dairy vanilla ice cream.

Lemon Blueberry Quinoa Cookies

Ingredients:

- 1 cup cooked quinoa, cooled
- 1/2 cup almond flour
- 1/4 cup coconut oil, melted
- 1/4 cup maple syrup
- Zest of one lemon
- 1/2 cup blueberries

Prep Time: 15 minutes

Cooking Time: 15 minutes

Serving Time: Immediate

Nutritional Info: High in fiber, healthy fats, and antioxidants

Instructions:

- Preheat the oven to 350°F (175°C).

- In a bowl, mix cooked quinoa, almond flour, melted coconut oil, maple syrup, lemon zest, and blueberries.
- Drop spoonsful of the mixture onto a baking sheet and bake until golden.

Serving Methods:

1. Drizzle with a lemon glaze for extra sweetness.
2. Serve with a cup of herbal tea for a delightful pairing.

Cinnamon Raisin Oatmeal Cookies

Ingredients:

- 1 cup rolled oats
- 1/2 cup almond flour
- 1/4 cup coconut oil, melted
- 1/4 cup maple syrup
- 1/2 teaspoon cinnamon
- 1/4 cup raisins

Prep Time: 15 minutes

Cooking Time: 12 minutes

Serving Time: Immediate

Nutritional Info: High in fiber, healthy fats, and antioxidants

Instructions:

- Preheat the oven to 350°F (175°C).

- In a bowl, combine rolled oats, almond flour, melted coconut oil, maple syrup, cinnamon, and raisins.
- Scoop spoonfuls of the mixture onto a baking sheet and bake until golden.

Serving Methods:

1. Sandwich with almond butter for a delightful treat.
2. Serve with a warm cup of herbal tea.

Berry and Chia Seed Parfait

Ingredients:

- 1 cup mixed berries (strawberries, blueberries, raspberries)
- 2 tablespoons chia seeds
- 1 cup coconut yogurt
- 1 tablespoon honey

Prep Time: 10 minutes

Setting Time: 2 hours (for chia seeds)

Serving Time: Immediate

Nutritional Info: High in fiber, antioxidants, and probiotics

Instructions:

- In a bowl, mix chia seeds with coconut yogurt and let it set for at least 2 hours.

- Layer chia seed mixture with mixed berries in serving glasses.
- Drizzle with honey before serving.

Serving Methods:

1. Top with a sprinkle of granola for added crunch.
2. Serve in small mason jars for a visually appealing presentation.

Dark Chocolate-Dipped Strawberries

Ingredients:

- 1 cup dark chocolate, melted
- 1 pint fresh strawberries, washed and dried

Prep Time: 10 minutes

Setting Time: 30 minutes (for chocolate to harden)

Serving Time: Immediate

Nutritional Info: High in antioxidants, vitamins, and minerals

Instructions:

- Dip each strawberry into melted dark chocolate, covering halfway.
- Place on a parchment-lined tray and let it set in the refrigerator for at least 30 minutes.

Serving Methods:

1. Sprinkle with crushed pistachios for added texture.

2. Serve with a side of mint leaves for a refreshing touch.

Mint Chocolate Avocado Mousse

Ingredients:

- 2 ripe avocados

- 1/4 cup unsweetened cocoa powder

- 1/4 cup maple syrup

- 1 teaspoon peppermint extract

Prep Time: 10 minutes

Setting Time: 1 hour (for chilling)

Serving Time: Immediate

Nutritional Info: High in healthy fats, antioxidants, and vitamins

Instructions:

- In a blender, combine ripe avocados, cocoa powder, maple syrup, and peppermint extract.

- Blend until smooth and creamy.

- Chill in the refrigerator for at least 1 hour before serving.

Serving Methods:

1. Top with dairy-free whipped cream for extra indulgence.

2. Serve in small cups for portion control.

Almond Flour Lemon Poppy Seed Muffins

Ingredients:

- 1 cup almond flour
- 1/4 cup coconut flour
- 1/4 cup coconut oil, melted
- 1/4 cup maple syrup
- Zest of one lemon
- 1 tablespoon poppy seeds

Prep Time: 15 minutes

Cooking Time: 20 minutes

Serving Time: Immediate

Nutritional Info: High in fiber, healthy fats, and vitamin C

Instructions:

- Preheat the oven to 350°F (175°C).
- In a bowl, mix almond flour, coconut flour, melted coconut oil, maple syrup, lemon zest, and poppy seeds.
- Spoon the batter into muffin cups and bake until golden.

Serving Methods:

1. Drizzle with a lemon glaze for extra sweetness.
2. Serve with a side of fresh berries for a delightful contrast.

Pineapple and Coconut Sorbet

Ingredients:

- 2 cups fresh pineapple, diced
- 1/2 cup coconut milk
- 2 tablespoons shredded coconut
- Mint leaves for garnish

Prep Time: 10 minutes

Freezing Time: 4 hours

Serving Time: Immediate

Nutritional Info: High in vitamins, antioxidants, and healthy fats

Instructions:

- In a blender, blend fresh pineapple and coconut milk until smooth.
- Transfer the mixture to a shallow dish, sprinkle with shredded coconut, and freeze for at least 4 hours.
- Scoop into bowls and garnish with mint leaves.

Serving Methods:

1. Drizzle with honey for a touch of sweetness.
2. Serve with a slice of grilled pineapple for added flair.

Raspberry Almond Thumbprint Cookies

Ingredients:

- 1 cup almond flour

- 1/4 cup coconut oil, melted
- 1/4 cup raspberry jam (no added sugar)

Prep Time: 10 minutes

Cooking Time: 12 minutes

Serving Time: Immediate

Nutritional Info: High in healthy fats, fiber, and antioxidants

Instructions:

- Preheat the oven to 350°F (175°C).
- In a bowl, mix almond flour and melted coconut oil.
- Form small balls of dough, make an indentation with your thumb, and fill with raspberry jam.
- Bake until edges are golden.

Serving Methods:

1. Dust with powdered sugar for a festive touch.
2. Serve with a cup of herbal tea for a comforting treat.

Turmeric Golden Milk Popsicles

Ingredients:

- 1 cup coconut milk
- 1 teaspoon turmeric powder
- 1/2 teaspoon ginger powder
- 2 tablespoons honey

Pinch of black pepper

Prep Time: 10 minutes

Freezing Time: 4 hours

Serving Time: Immediate

Nutritional Info: High in antioxidants, anti-inflammatory properties, and vitamins

Instructions:

- In a bowl, whisk together coconut milk, turmeric powder, ginger powder, honey, and black pepper.
- Pour into popsicle molds and freeze for at least 4 hours.
- Remove from molds and enjoy.

Serving Methods:

1. Roll in crushed pistachios for added crunch.
2. Serve with a sprinkle of ground cinnamon for extra flavor.

Fig and Walnut Energy Bites

Ingredients:

- 1 cup dried figs, soaked
- 1 cup walnuts
- 1/4 cup coconut flour
- 1 tablespoon chia seeds

Prep Time: 15 minutes

Setting Time: 30 minutes (for chilling)

Serving Time: Immediate

Nutritional Info: High in fiber, healthy fats, and protein

Instructions:

- In a food processor, blend soaked figs, walnuts, coconut flour, and chia seeds until a dough-like consistency forms.
- Roll into bite-sized balls and chill in the refrigerator for 30 minutes.

Serving Methods:

1. Dust with cocoa powder for a chocolatey touch.
2. Serve with a side of Greek yogurt for added richness.

Peach and Almond Crisp

Ingredients:

- 3 cups sliced peaches
- 1/2 cup almond flour
- 1/4 cup coconut oil, melted
- 2 tablespoons maple syrup
- 1/2 teaspoon cinnamon

Prep Time: 15 minutes

Cooking Time: 30 minutes

Serving Time: Immediate

Nutritional Info: High in fiber, healthy fats, and vitamins

Instructions:

- Preheat the oven to 375°F (190°C).
- In a bowl, mix sliced peaches with almond flour, melted coconut oil, maple syrup, and cinnamon.
- Transfer to a baking dish and bake until the top is golden and bubbly.

Serving Methods:

1. Top with a scoop of vanilla coconut ice cream.
2. Serve warm with a sprinkle of sliced almonds for added crunch

CHAPTER EIGHT

SALAD RECIPES

Mediterranean Quinoa Salad

Ingredients:

- 1 cup cooked quinoa
- Cherry tomatoes, halved
- Cucumber, diced
- Kalamata olives, pitted
- Red onion, thinly sliced
- Feta cheese, crumbled
- Fresh parsley, chopped

Prep Time: 15 minutes

Serving Time: Immediate

Nutritional Info: High in fiber, protein, and antioxidants

Instructions:

- In a bowl, combine cooked quinoa, cherry tomatoes, cucumber, olives, red onion, and feta cheese.
- Sprinkle with fresh parsley.
- Drizzle with olive oil and lemon juice.

Serving Methods:

1. Serve as a side dish with grilled chicken.

2. Wrap in collard green leaves for a portable option.

Kale and Avocado Salad with Lemon Tahini Dressing

Ingredients:

- Fresh kale, stems removed and chopped
- Avocado, sliced
- Carrot, shredded
- Red cabbage, thinly sliced
- Sunflower seeds
- Lemon Tahini Dressing (tahini, lemon juice, olive oil)

Prep Time: 10 minutes

Serving Time: Immediate

Nutritional Info: High in vitamins, healthy fats, and fiber

Instructions:

- Massage kale with a bit of olive oil to soften.
- Toss kale with avocado, shredded carrot, red cabbage, and sunflower seeds.
- Drizzle with Lemon Tahini Dressing.

Serving Methods:

1. Top with grilled salmon for added protein.
2. Serve with a side of quinoa for a complete meal.

Asian-Inspired Edamame Salad

Ingredients:

- Edamame, cooked and shelled
- Red bell pepper, julienned
- Shredded cabbage
- Carrot, thinly sliced
- Sesame seeds
- Ginger-Soy Dressing (soy sauce, sesame oil, ginger)

Prep Time: 15 minutes

Serving Time: Immediate

Nutritional Info: High in protein, vitamins, and antioxidants

Instructions:

- In a bowl, combine edamame, red bell pepper, shredded cabbage, and carrot.
- Sprinkle with sesame seeds.
- Toss with Ginger-Soy Dressing.

Serving Methods:

1. Top with grilled tofu for a vegetarian option.
2. Serve over a bed of brown rice for a heartier dish.

Spinach and Strawberry Salad with Balsamic Vinaigrette

Ingredients:

- Fresh spinach leaves
- Strawberries, sliced
- Goat cheese, crumbled
- Walnuts, chopped
- Balsamic Vinaigrette (balsamic vinegar, olive oil, Dijon mustard)

Prep Time: 10 minutes

Serving Time: Immediate

Nutritional Info: High in antioxidants, vitamins, and healthy fats

Instructions:

- In a salad bowl, combine fresh spinach, sliced strawberries, crumbled goat cheese, and chopped walnuts.
- Toss with Balsamic Vinaigrette.

Serving Methods:

Top with grilled chicken or shrimp for added protein.

Serve as a refreshing side with a bowl of vegetable soup.

Cauliflower Tabbouleh Salad

Ingredients:

- Cauliflower, grated
- Cherry tomatoes, diced
- Cucumber, finely chopped
- Fresh mint, chopped
- Red onion, minced
- Lemon juice and olive oil dressing

Prep Time: 15 minutes

Serving Time: Immediate

Nutritional Info: Low-carb, high in vitamins, and antioxidants

Instructions:

- Grate cauliflower into a tabbouleh-like consistency.
- Combine with cherry tomatoes, cucumber, fresh mint, and red onion.
- Dress with a mixture of lemon juice and olive oil.

Serving Methods:

1. Serve as a light lunch with a side of hummus.
2. Wrap in lettuce leaves for a low-carb alternative.

Tuna and Chickpea Salad

Ingredients:

- Canned tuna, drained
- Chickpeas, rinsed and drained

- Cherry tomatoes, halved
- Cucumber, diced
- Red bell pepper, chopped
- Feta cheese, crumbled
- Lemon herb dressing (lemon juice, olive oil, herbs)

Prep Time: 15 minutes

Serving Time: Immediate

Nutritional Info: High in protein, fiber, and omega-3s

Instructions

- In a large bowl, mix tuna, chickpeas, cherry tomatoes, cucumber, red bell pepper, and feta cheese.
- Toss with Lemon Herb Dressing.

Serving Methods:

1. Spoon over a bed of mixed greens for a main course.
2. Serve in whole-grain pita pockets for a portable option.

Roasted Vegetable Quinoa Salad

Ingredients:

- Quinoa, cooked
- Zucchini, diced
- Cherry tomatoes, halved
- Red onion, sliced

- Bell peppers, chopped
- Fresh basil, chopped
- Balsamic vinaigrette (balsamic vinegar, olive oil, garlic)

Prep Time: 20 minutes

Cooking Time: 20 minutes (for roasting)

Serving Time: Immediate

Nutritional Info: High in fiber, vitamins, and antioxidants

Instructions:

- Roast zucchini, cherry tomatoes, red onion, and bell peppers in the oven.
- In a bowl, combine cooked quinoa with the roasted vegetables.
- Toss with Balsamic Vinaigrette and garnish with fresh basil.

Serving Methods:

1. Top with grilled chicken or salmon for added protein.
2. Serve as a side dish with a piece of crusty whole-grain bread.

Beet and Goat Cheese Salad with Honey Mustard Dressing

Ingredients:

- Roasted beets, sliced

- Mixed greens

- Goat cheese, crumbled

- Candied pecans

- Honey Mustard Dressing (honey, Dijon mustard, olive oil)

Prep Time: 15 minutes

Cooking Time: 45 minutes (for roasting beets)

Serving Time: Immediate

Nutritional Info: High in fiber, antioxidants, and healthy fats

Instructions:

- Roast beets in the oven and let them cool before slicing.

- In a salad bowl, combine mixed greens, sliced beets, crumbled goat cheese, and candied pecans.

- Drizzle with Honey Mustard Dressing.

Serving Methods:

1. Serve alongside a grilled turkey or chicken breast.
2. Pair with a cup of vegetable soup for a light lunch.

Greek Cucumber Salad

Ingredients:

- English cucumbers, diced

- Cherry tomatoes, halved
- Kalamata olives, pitted
- Red onion, thinly sliced
- Feta cheese, crumbled
- Greek dressing (olive oil, red wine vinegar, oregano)

Prep Time: 10 minutes

Serving Time: Immediate

Nutritional Info: High in vitamins, healthy fats, and antioxidants

Instructions:

- In a bowl, combine diced cucumbers, cherry tomatoes, olives, red onion, and feta cheese.
- Toss with Greek dressing.

Serving Methods:

- Serve as a side dish with grilled fish or shrimp.
- Spoon over whole-grain couscous for a Mediterranean-inspired meal.

Orange and Arugula Salad with Citrus Vinaigrette

Ingredients:

- Arugula
- Oranges, peeled and segmented

- Red onion, thinly sliced
- Goat cheese, crumbled
- Almonds, sliced
- Citrus Vinaigrette (orange juice, lemon juice, olive oil)

Prep Time: 15 minutes

Serving Time: Immediate

Nutritional Info: High in vitamins, antioxidants, and healthy fats

Instructions:

- In a large salad bowl, combine arugula, orange segments, red onion, crumbled goat cheese, and sliced almonds.
- Drizzle with Citrus Vinaigrette.

Serving Methods:

1. Top with grilled chicken or tofu for a protein boost.
2. Serve with a side of whole-grain quinoa for a complete meal.

Broccoli and Cranberry Salad

Ingredients:

- Broccoli florets, blanched
- Dried cranberries

- Red onion, finely chopped
- Sunflower seeds
- Greek yogurt dressing (Greek yogurt, honey, Dijon mustard)

Prep Time: 15 minutes

Serving Time: Immediate

Nutritional Info: High in fiber, vitamins, and antioxidants

Instructions:

- In a bowl, combine blanched broccoli, dried cranberries, red onion, and sunflower seeds.
- Toss with Greek yogurt dressing.

Serving Methods:

1. Add grilled chicken or turkey for a protein-packed meal.
2. Serve on a bed of mixed greens for added freshness.

Caprese Salad Skewers

Ingredients:

- Cherry tomatoes
- Fresh mozzarella balls
- Basil leaves
- Balsamic glaze
- Olive oil

- Sea salt and black pepper

Prep Time: 10 minutes

Serving Time: Immediate

Nutritional Info: High in calcium, vitamins, and healthy fats

Instructions:

- Thread cherry tomatoes, fresh mozzarella balls, and basil leaves onto skewers.
- Drizzle with balsamic glaze and olive oil.
- Sprinkle with sea salt and black pepper.

Serving Methods:

1. Serve as an elegant appetizer for gatherings.
2. Arrange on a plate with mixed greens for a light lunch.

Warm Brussels Sprouts Salad

Ingredients:

- Brussels sprouts, halved
- Pomegranate seeds
- Toasted pecans, chopped
- Feta cheese, crumbled
- Maple Dijon dressing (maple syrup, Dijon mustard, apple cider vinegar)

Prep Time: 20 minutes

Cooking Time: 15 minutes

Serving Time: Immediate

Nutritional Info: High in fiber, antioxidants, and healthy fats

Instructions:

- Roast Brussels sprouts until golden and slightly crispy.
- In a bowl, combine roasted Brussels sprouts, pomegranate seeds, toasted pecans, and feta cheese.
- Toss with Maple Dijon dressing.

Serving Methods:

1. Top with grilled chicken or salmon for added protein.
2. Serve warm as a comforting side dish.

Cabbage and Apple Slaw

Ingredients:

- Red cabbage, thinly sliced
- Green apples, julienned
- Carrots, shredded
- Raisins
- Greek yogurt coleslaw dressing (Greek yogurt, apple cider vinegar, honey)

Prep Time: 15 minutes

Serving Time: Immediate

Nutritional Info: High in fiber, vitamins, and antioxidants

Instructions:

- In a large bowl, combine sliced red cabbage, julienned green apples, shredded carrots, and raisins.
- Toss with Greek yogurt coleslaw dressing.

Serving Methods:

1. Add grilled turkey or chicken for a protein boost.
2. Serve as a side dish at barbecues or picnics.

Chickpea and Avocado Salad

Ingredients:

- Canned chickpeas, rinsed and drained
- Avocado, diced
- Cherry tomatoes, halved
- Cucumber, diced
- Red onion, finely chopped
- Cilantro, chopped
- Lime vinaigrette (lime juice, olive oil, garlic)

Prep Time: 15 minutes

Serving Time: Immediate

Nutritional Info: High in protein, healthy fats, and vitamins

Instructions:

- In a bowl, mix chickpeas, diced avocado, cherry tomatoes, cucumber, red onion, and cilantro.
- Toss with Lime Vinaigrette.

Serving Methods:

1. Spoon onto whole-grain wraps for a portable lunch.
2. Top with grilled shrimp or fish for a complete meal.

Mango and Black Bean Quinoa Salad

ance*Ingredients:*

- Cooked quinoa
- Black beans, canned and rinsed
- Mango, diced
- Red bell pepper, chopped
- Red onion, minced
- Cilantro, chopped
- Lime dressing (lime juice, olive oil, cumin)

Prep Time: 20 minutes

Serving Time: Immediate

Nutritional Info: High in fiber, protein, and vitamins

Instructions:

- In a large bowl, combine cooked quinoa, black beans, diced mango, chopped red bell pepper, minced red onion, and cilantro.
- Toss with Lime Dressing.

Serving Methods:

1. Serve chilled as a refreshing summer salad.
2. Top with grilled chicken or tofu for added protein.

Pesto Pasta Salad with Cherry Tomatoes and Pine Nuts

Ingredients:

- Whole-grain pasta, cooked
- Cherry tomatoes, halved
- Fresh mozzarella balls, halved
- Pine nuts, toasted
- Fresh basil pesto (basil, pine nuts, garlic, olive oil)

Prep Time: 20 minutes

Cooking Time: 10 minutes (for pasta)

Serving Time: Immediate

Nutritional Info: High in fiber, calcium, and healthy fats

Instructions:

- Cook whole-grain pasta according to package instructions and let it cool.
- In a bowl, toss pasta with cherry tomatoes, fresh mozzarella, toasted pine nuts, and fresh basil pesto.

Serving Methods:

1. Serve as a side dish at summer gatherings or barbecues.
2. Pack for a picnic or outdoor lunch.

Cucumber and Dill Greek Salad

Ingredients:

- English cucumbers, diced
- Cherry tomatoes, halved
- Feta cheese, crumbled
- Kalamata olives, pitted
- Fresh dill, chopped
- Greek dressing (olive oil, red wine vinegar, oregano)

Prep Time: 10 minutes

Serving Time: Immediate

Nutritional Info: High in vitamins, healthy fats, and antioxidants

Instructions:

- In a salad bowl, combine diced cucumbers, cherry tomatoes, crumbled feta cheese, pitted Kalamata olives, and chopped fresh dill.
- Toss with Greek dressing.

Serving Methods:

1. Serve as a refreshing side with grilled lamb or chicken.
2. Spoon onto whole-grain pita bread for a light lunch.

Spicy Mango Chicken Salad

Ingredients:

- Grilled chicken breast, sliced
- Romaine lettuce, chopped
- Mango, diced
- Red bell pepper, thinly sliced
- Jalapeño, finely chopped
- Cilantro, chopped
- Lime-chili dressing (lime juice, chili powder, olive oil)

Prep Time: 15 minutes

Cooking Time: 15 minutes (for grilling chicken)

Serving Time: Immediate

Nutritional Info: High in protein, vitamins, and antioxidants

Instructions:

- Grill chicken breast until fully cooked and slice.
- In a large bowl, combine chopped romaine lettuce, diced mango, sliced red bell pepper, chopped jalapeño, and cilantro.
- Toss with Lime-Chili Dressing.

Serving Methods:

1. Top with avocado slices for added creaminess.
2. Serve as a main course for a light dinner.

Peach and Arugula Salad with Balsamic Reduction

Ingredients:

- Arugula
- Fresh peaches, sliced
- Goat cheese, crumbled
- Pecans, toasted and chopped
- Balsamic reduction

Prep Time: 15 minutes

Serving Time: Immediate

Nutritional Info: High in vitamins, antioxidants, and healthy fats

Instructions:

- In a large salad bowl, combine arugula, sliced peaches, crumbled goat cheese, and chopped pecans.
- Drizzle with balsamic reduction.

Serving Methods:

1. Top with grilled chicken or salmon for added protein.
2. Serve as a side dish at summer gatherings.

CHAPTER EIGHT

SOUP RECIPES

Vegetable Quinoa Soup

Ingredients:

- 1 cup quinoa, rinsed
- Mixed vegetables (carrots, celery, zucchini), diced
- Kale, chopped
- Vegetable broth
- Garlic, minced
- Fresh thyme
- Olive oil
- Salt and pepper to taste

Prep Time: 15 minutes

Cooking Time: 30 minutes

Serving Time: Immediate

Nutritional Info: High in fiber, vitamins, and minerals

Instructions:

- In a large pot, sauté garlic in olive oil until fragrant.
- Add mixed vegetables and kale, sauté until slightly softened.
- Pour in vegetable broth, add quinoa and fresh thyme.

- Simmer until quinoa is cooked, season with salt and pepper.

Serving Methods:

1. Serve with a sprinkle of nutritional yeast for added flavor.
2. Pair with a slice of whole-grain bread.

Miso Mushroom Soup

Ingredients:

- 4 cups vegetable broth
- 1 cup mushrooms, sliced
- Tofu, cubed
- Wakame seaweed, soaked
- 3 tablespoons miso paste
- Green onions, sliced
- Sesame oil

Prep Time: 10 minutes

Cooking Time: 15 minutes

Serving Time: Immediate

Nutritional Info: High in antioxidants, probiotics, and vitamins

Instructions:

- Bring vegetable broth to a simmer, add mushrooms, tofu, and soaked Wakame seaweed.

- In a small bowl, dissolve miso paste in a bit of broth and add to the pot.
- Stir well, garnish with green onions, and drizzle with sesame oil.

Serving Methods:

1. Serve as an appetizer before a meal.
2. Pair with a side of steamed brown rice.

Lentil and Vegetable Soup

Ingredients:

- 1 cup dried lentils, rinsed
- Carrots, celery, and onion, diced
- Spinach, chopped
- Vegetable broth
- Garlic, minced
- Cumin and coriander for seasoning
- Olive oil
- Lemon wedges for serving

Prep Time: 20 minutes

Cooking Time: 45 minutes

Serving Time: Immediate

Nutritional Info: High in fiber, protein, and vitamins

Instructions:

- Sauté garlic, carrots, celery, and onion in olive oil until softened.
- Add lentils, vegetable broth, cumin, and coriander.
- Simmer until lentils are tender, stir in chopped spinach.
- Serve with a squeeze of lemon.

Serving Methods:

1. Pair with a side of quinoa for added protein.
2. Top with a dollop of Greek yogurt for creaminess.

Butternut Squash and Apple Soup

Ingredients:

- 1 medium butternut squash, peeled and cubed
- Apples, peeled and diced
- Onion, chopped
- Vegetable broth
- Ginger, grated
- Coconut milk
- Cinnamon for seasoning
- Olive oil

Prep Time: 15 minutes

Cooking Time: 30 minutes

Serving Time: Immediate

Nutritional Info: High in vitamins, antioxidants, and fiber

Instructions:

- Sauté onions in olive oil until translucent, add butternut squash and apples.
- Pour in vegetable broth, add grated ginger, and simmer until squash is tender.
- Blend until smooth, stir in coconut milk and season with cinnamon.

Serving Methods:

1. Garnish with toasted pumpkin seeds for texture.
2. Serve with a side of whole-grain crackers.

Tomato Basil Quinoa Soup

Ingredients:

- 2 cups cherry tomatoes, halved
- Quinoa, rinsed
- Vegetable broth
- Onion, diced
- Garlic, minced
- Fresh basil, chopped
- Olive oil
- Salt and pepper to taste

Prep Time: 15 minutes

Cooking Time: 25 minutes

Serving Time: Immediate

Nutritional Info: High in antioxidants, fiber, and vitamins

Instructions:

- Sauté onions and garlic in olive oil until softened.
- Add cherry tomatoes, quinoa, and vegetable broth.
- Simmer until quinoa is cooked, stir in fresh basil, and season with salt and pepper.

Serving Methods:

1. Top with a swirl of balsamic reduction for added flavor.
2. Serve with a side of mixed green salad.

Spinach and Chickpea Lemon Soup

Ingredients:

- 1 can chickpeas, rinsed and drained
- Spinach, chopped
- Vegetable broth
- Lemon juice
- Garlic, minced
- Cumin and paprika for seasoning
- Olive oil

Prep Time: 15 minutes

Cooking Time: 20 minutes

Serving Time: Immediate

Nutritional Info: High in protein, vitamins, and antioxidants

Instructions:

- Sauté garlic in olive oil until fragrant.
- Add chickpeas, vegetable broth, cumin, and paprika.
- Simmer until chickpeas are tender, stir in chopped spinach.
- Finish with a squeeze of fresh lemon juice.

Serving Methods:

1. Serve over a bed of cooked quinoa for a complete meal.
2. Garnish with a sprinkle of nutritional yeast.

Carrot Ginger Turmeric Soup

Ingredients:

- Carrots, chopped
- Ginger, grated
- Turmeric powder
- Vegetable broth
- Coconut milk
- Onion, diced
- Garlic, minced
- Olive oil

Prep Time: 15 minutes

Cooking Time: 30 minutes

Nutritional Info: High in antioxidants, anti-inflammatory properties, and vitamins

Instructions:

- Sauté onions and garlic in olive oil until softened.
- Add chopped carrots, grated ginger, turmeric, and vegetable broth.
- Simmer until carrots are tender, blend until smooth, and stir in coconut milk.

Serving Methods:

1. Drizzle with a swirl of coconut cream for richness.
2. Serve with a side of whole-grain naan bread.

Cauliflower Leek Soup

Ingredients:

- Cauliflower, chopped
- Leeks, sliced
- Vegetable broth
- Almond milk
- Garlic, minced
- Nutmeg for seasoning
- Olive oil

Prep Time: 20 minutes

Cooking Time: 25 minutes

Serving Time: Immediate

Nutritional Info: Low in calories, high in vitamins and minerals

Instructions:

- Sauté leeks and garlic in olive oil until softened.
- Add chopped cauliflower, vegetable broth, and nutmeg.
- Simmer until cauliflower is tender, blend until smooth, and stir in almond milk.

Serving Methods:

1. Garnish with chopped chives for freshness.
2. Serve with a side of roasted chickpeas for added crunch.

Kale and White Bean Soup

Ingredients:

- Cannellini beans, canned and rinsed
- Kale, chopped
- Vegetable broth
- Tomatoes, diced
- Onion, diced
- Garlic, minced
- Italian seasoning
- Olive oil

Prep Time: 15 minutes

Cooking Time: 25 minutes

Serving Time: Immediate

Nutritional Info: High in fiber, protein, and vitamins

Instructions:

- Sauté onions and garlic in olive oil until softened.
- Add diced tomatoes, cannellini beans, vegetable broth, and Italian seasoning.
- Simmer until flavors meld, stir in chopped kale.

Serving Methods:

1. Top with a drizzle of extra virgin olive oil for richness.
2. Serve with a side of whole-grain crusty bread.

Sweet Potato and Coconut Curry Soup

Ingredients:

- Sweet potatoes, peeled and diced
- Coconut milk
- Red curry paste
- Vegetable broth
- Onion, chopped
- Garlic, minced
- Lime juice
- Olive oil

Prep Time: 20 minutes

Cooking Time: 30 minutes

Serving Time: Immediate

Nutritional Info: High in vitamins, antioxidants, and healthy fats

Instructions:

- Sauté onions and garlic in olive oil until softened.
- Add diced sweet potatoes, red curry paste, and vegetable broth.
- Simmer until sweet potatoes are tender, stir in coconut milk, and finish with a squeeze of lime juice.

Serving Methods:

1. Garnish with chopped cilantro for freshness.
2. Serve over a bed of brown rice for a hearty option

Barley and Vegetable Soup

Ingredients:

- Pearl barley, rinsed
- Mixed vegetables (carrots, celery, peas), diced
- Vegetable broth
- Onion, diced
- Garlic, minced
- Thyme and rosemary for seasoning
- Olive oil

Prep Time: 15 minutes

Cooking Time: 45 minutes

Serving Time: Immediate

Nutritional Info: High in fiber, vitamins, and minerals

Instructions:

- Sauté onions and garlic in olive oil until softened.
- Add mixed vegetables, vegetable broth, pearl barley, and herbs.
- Simmer until barley is cooked, season with salt and pepper.

Serving Methods:

1. Top with a dollop of Greek yogurt for added creaminess.
2. Serve with a side of whole-grain bread.

Red Lentil and Spinach Soup

Ingredients:

- Red lentils, rinsed
- Spinach, chopped
- Vegetable broth
- Tomatoes, diced
- Onion, chopped
- Cumin and coriander for seasoning
- Garlic, minced
- Olive oil

Prep Time: 15 minutes

Cooking Time: 30 minutes

Serving Time: Immediate

Nutritional Info: High in protein, fiber, and vitamins

Instructions:

- Sauté onions and garlic in olive oil until softened.
- Add diced tomatoes, red lentils, vegetable broth, cumin, and coriander.
- Simmer until lentils are tender, stir in chopped spinach.

Serving Methods:

1. Garnish with a swirl of coconut cream for richness.
2. Serve with a side of quinoa for added protein.

Cabbage and Chickpea Stew

Ingredients:

- Cabbage, shredded
- Chickpeas, cooked
- Tomatoes, diced
- Vegetable broth
- Onion, diced
- Paprika and oregano for seasoning
- Garlic, minced
- Olive oil

Prep Time: 20 minutes

Cooking Time: 30 minutes

Serving Time: Immediate

Nutritional Info: High in fiber, protein, and vitamins

Instructions:

- Sauté onions and garlic in olive oil until softened.
- Add shredded cabbage, diced tomatoes, chickpeas, vegetable broth, paprika, and oregano.
- Simmer until cabbage is tender, season with salt and pepper.

Serving Methods:

1. Top with a spoonful of plain Greek yogurt for creaminess.
2. Serve over a bed of brown rice for a wholesome meal.

Zucchini and Basil Soup

Ingredients:

- Zucchini, sliced
- Basil leaves, chopped
- Vegetable broth
- Onion, diced
- Garlic, minced
- Lemon zest
- Olive oil

- Salt and pepper to taste

Prep Time: 15 minutes

Cooking Time: 25 minutes

Serving Time: Immediate

Nutritional Info: Low-calorie, high in vitamins, and antioxidants

Instructions:

- Sauté onions and garlic in olive oil until softened.
- Add sliced zucchini, vegetable broth, and chopped basil.
- Simmer until zucchini is tender, season with lemon zest, salt, and pepper.

Serving Methods:

1. Drizzle with a touch of extra virgin olive oil for richness.
2. Serve with a side of whole-grain crackers.

Cauliflower and Broccoli Soup

Ingredients:

- Cauliflower, chopped
- Broccoli florets
- Vegetable broth
- Onion, diced
- Garlic, minced
- Nutmeg and thyme for seasoning
- Almond milk

- Olive oil

Prep Time: 20 minutes

Cooking Time: 30 minutes

Serving Time: Immediate

Nutritional Info: Low-calorie, high in vitamins, and minerals

Instructions:

- Sauté onions and garlic in olive oil until softened.
- Add chopped cauliflower, broccoli, vegetable broth, nutmeg, and thyme.
- Simmer until vegetables are tender, blend until smooth, and stir in almond milk.

Serving Methods:

1. Garnish with a sprinkle of chopped chives for freshness.
2. Serve with a side of whole-grain toast.

Spiced Pumpkin Soup

Ingredients:

- Pumpkin, peeled and diced
- Coconut milk
- Vegetable broth
- Onion, chopped
- Garlic, minced
- Curry powder and cayenne for seasoning

- Olive oil

Prep Time: 15 minutes

Cooking Time: 25 minutes

Serving Time: Immediate

Nutritional Info: High in vitamins, antioxidants, and healthy fats

Instructions:

- Sauté onions and garlic in olive oil until softened.
- Add diced pumpkin, vegetable broth, coconut milk, curry powder, and cayenne.
- Simmer until pumpkin is tender, blend until smooth.

Serving Methods:

1. Swirl with a touch of coconut cream for added richness.
2. Serve with a side of quinoa for a complete meal.

Wild Rice and Mushroom Soup

Ingredients:

- Wild rice, cooked
- Mushrooms, sliced
- Vegetable broth
- Celery, diced
- Onion, chopped
- Thyme and sage for seasoning
- Garlic, minced

- Olive oil

Prep Time: 20 minutes

Cooking Time: 45 minutes

Serving Time: Immediate

Nutritional Info: High in fiber, protein, and vitamins

Instructions:

- Sauté onions and garlic in olive oil until softened.
- Add sliced mushrooms, diced celery, vegetable broth, thyme, and sage.
- Simmer until vegetables are tender, stir in cooked wild rice.

Serving Methods:

1. Garnish with a sprinkle of chopped parsley for freshness.
2. Serve with a side of crusty whole-grain bread.

Tomato and Lentil Soup

Ingredients:

- Red lentils, rinsed
- Tomatoes, diced
- Vegetable broth
- Onion, chopped
- Garlic, minced
- Basil and oregano for seasoning

- Olive oil

Prep Time: 15 minutes

Cooking Time: 30 minutes

Serving Time: Immediate

Nutritional Info: High in protein, vitamins, and antioxidants

Instructions:

- Sauté onions and garlic in olive oil until softened.
- Add diced tomatoes, red lentils, vegetable broth, basil, and oregano.
- Simmer until lentils are tender, season with salt and pepper.

Serving Methods:

1. Top with a dollop of pesto for added flavor.
2. Serve with a side of whole-grain garlic bread.

Brussels Sprouts and Potato Chowder

Ingredients:

- Brussels sprouts, halved
- Potatoes, diced
- Vegetable broth
- Onion, diced
- Garlic, minced
- Thyme and rosemary for seasoning

- Almond milk
- Olive oil

Prep Time: 20 minutes

Cooking Time: 30 minutes

Serving Time: Immediate

Nutritional Info: High in fiber, vitamins, and minerals

Instructions:

- Sauté onions and garlic in olive oil until softened.
- Add halved Brussels sprouts, diced potatoes, vegetable broth, thyme, and rosemary.
- Simmer until vegetables are tender, stir in almond milk.

Serving Methods:

1. Garnish with a sprinkle of nutritional yeast for added flavor.
2. Serve with a side of whole-grain crackers.

Lemon Chickpea Orzo Soup

Ingredients:

- Orzo pasta, cooked
- Chickpeas, cooked
- Vegetable broth
- Spinach, chopped
- Lemon juice

- Onion, diced
- Garlic, minced
- Dill for seasoning
- Olive oil

Prep Time: 15 minutes

Cooking Time: 20 minutes

Serving Time: Immediate

Nutritional Info: High in protein, vitamins, and antioxidants

Instructions:

- Sauté onions and garlic in olive oil until softened.
- Add cooked orzo, chickpeas, vegetable broth, chopped spinach, and dill.
- Simmer until spinach is wilted, finish with a squeeze of fresh lemon juice.

Serving Methods:

1. Top with a swirl of Greek yogurt for creaminess.
2. Serve with a side of whole-grain pita bread.

CHAPTER EIGHT

MEAT AND POULTRY RECIPES

Grilled Lemon Herb Chicken

Ingredients:

- Chicken breasts
- Lemon juice
- Fresh thyme and rosemary
- Garlic, minced
- Olive oil
- Salt and pepper to taste

Prep Time: 15 minutes

Cooking Time: 20 minutes

Serving Time: Immediate

Nutritional Info: High in protein, vitamins, and antioxidants

Instructions:

- Marinate chicken in a mixture of lemon juice, minced garlic, fresh thyme, rosemary, olive oil, salt, and pepper.
- Grill until fully cooked.
- Serve with a side of roasted vegetables or a quinoa salad.

Serving Methods:

1. Slice and serve over a bed of mixed greens for a refreshing salad.

2. Pair with sweet potato wedges for a satisfying meal.

Turkey and Vegetable Skewers

Ingredients:

- Ground turkey
- Bell peppers, onions, and cherry tomatoes
- Olive oil
- Cumin and paprika for seasoning
- Garlic, minced

Prep Time: 20 minutes

Cooking Time: 15 minutes

Serving Time: Immediate

Nutritional Info: High in protein, fiber, and vitamins

Instructions:

- Mix ground turkey with minced garlic, cumin, paprika, and olive oil.
- Form into small meatballs and thread onto skewers with veggies.
- Grill until turkey is cooked through.
- Serve with a side of quinoa or cauliflower rice.

Serving Methods:

1. Serve over a bed of sautéed spinach for a light dinner.
2. Accompany with a dipping sauce made with yogurt and herbs.

Baked Salmon with Dill Sauce

Ingredients:

- Salmon fillets
- Fresh dill, chopped
- Lemon juice
- Greek yogurt
- Dijon mustard
- Garlic, minced

Prep Time: 10 minutes

Cooking Time: 15 minutes

Serving Time: Immediate

Nutritional Info: High in omega-3 fatty acids, vitamins, and probiotics

Instructions:

- Mix chopped dill, lemon juice, Greek yogurt, Dijon mustard, and minced garlic to make the sauce.
- Brush salmon fillets with the sauce and bake until cooked.

- Serve with steamed asparagus or a quinoa salad.

Serving Methods:

1. Flake the salmon and serve in lettuce wraps for a light lunch.
2. Pair with a side of roasted sweet potatoes for a hearty dinner.

Lemon Herb Grilled Shrimp

Ingredients:

- Shrimp, peeled and deveined
- Lemon zest and juice
- Fresh parsley, chopped
- Olive oil
- Garlic, minced
- Salt and pepper to taste

Prep Time: 15 minutes

Cooking Time: 5 minutes

Serving Time: Immediate

Nutritional Info: High in protein, vitamins, and antioxidants

Instructions:

- Marinate shrimp in a mixture of lemon zest, lemon juice, chopped parsley, minced garlic, olive oil, salt, and pepper.
- Grill shrimp until they turn pink.
- Serve over a bed of quinoa or with a side of sautéed vegetables.

Serving Methods:

1. Toss grilled shrimp into a Mediterranean salad.
2. Skewer shrimp with cherry tomatoes for a delightful appetizer.

Balsamic Glazed Chicken Thighs

Ingredients:

- Chicken thighs, bone-in and skin-on
- Balsamic vinegar
- Honey
- Rosemary, chopped
- Garlic, minced
- Olive oil

Prep Time: 15 minutes

Cooking Time: 40 minutes

Serving Time: Immediate

Nutritional Info: High in protein, vitamins, and antioxidants

Instructions:

- Mix balsamic vinegar, honey, chopped rosemary, minced garlic, and olive oil to make the glaze.
- Coat chicken thighs with the glaze and bake until golden.
- Serve with roasted Brussels sprouts or a green bean almondine.

Serving Methods:

1. Shred leftover chicken and use it in wraps or sandwiches.
2. Pair with a side of quinoa for a balanced meal.

Stuffed Bell Peppers with Ground Turkey

Ingredients:

- Bell peppers, halved
- Ground turkey
- Quinoa, cooked
- Tomato sauce
- Onion, diced
- Italian seasoning
- Garlic, minced

Prep Time: 20 minutes

Cooking Time: 40 minutes

Serving Time: Immediate

Nutritional Info: High in protein, fiber, and vitamins

Instructions:

- Sauté ground turkey with diced onions, garlic, and Italian seasoning until cooked.
- Mix cooked quinoa and tomato sauce into the turkey mixture.
- Fill bell pepper halves with the turkey and quinoa mixture and bake until peppers are tender.

Serving Methods:

1. Top with a dollop of Greek yogurt for extra creaminess.
2. Serve over a bed of leafy greens for a light dinner.

Rosemary Lemon Grilled Chicken

Ingredients:

- Chicken drumsticks
- Lemon juice and zest
- Fresh rosemary, chopped
- Garlic, minced
- Olive oil
- Salt and pepper to taste

Prep Time: 15 minutes

Cooking Time: 30 minutes

Serving Time: Immediate

Nutritional Info: High in protein, vitamins, and antioxidants

Instructions:

- Marinate chicken drumsticks in lemon juice, lemon zest, chopped rosemary, minced garlic, olive oil, salt, and pepper.
- Grill until chicken is cooked through.
- Serve with a side of roasted sweet potatoes or a green salad.

Serving Methods:

1. Shred leftover chicken and use it in wraps or salads.
2. Serve with a side of quinoa for a well-rounded meal.

Garlic Herb Baked Turkey Breast

Ingredients:

- Turkey breast
- Garlic, minced
- Fresh thyme and sage, chopped
- Olive oil
- Lemon juice
- Salt and pepper to taste

Prep Time: 15 minutes

Cooking Time: 1 hour

Serving Time: Immediate

Nutritional Info: High in protein, vitamins, and antioxidants

Instructions:

- Rub turkey breast with minced garlic, chopped thyme, sage, olive oil, lemon juice, salt, and pepper.
- Bake until the turkey is cooked through and golden.
- Serve with a side of steamed broccoli or a wild rice pilaf.

Serving Methods:

1. Slice and use leftover turkey in sandwiches or wraps.
2. Serve with a side of quinoa for a nutritious meal.

Honey Mustard Glazed Salmon

Ingredients:

- Salmon fillets
- Dijon mustard
- Honey
- Lemon juice
- Olive oil
- Garlic, minced
- Fresh dill, chopped

Prep Time: 15 minutes

Cooking Time: 15 minutes

Serving Time: Immediate

Nutritional Info: High in omega-3 fatty acids, vitamins, and antioxidants

Instructions:

- Mix Dijon mustard, honey, lemon juice, minced garlic, and chopped dill to make the glaze.
- Coat salmon fillets with the glaze and bake until salmon is cooked.
- Serve with a side of quinoa or sautéed kale.

Serving Methods:

1. Flake leftover salmon and toss into a whole-grain pasta salad.
2. Serve with a side of roasted sweet potatoes for a filling dinner.

Mediterranean Chicken Kebabs

Ingredients:

- Chicken thighs, cubed
- Cherry tomatoes, olives, and red onion, threaded on skewers
- Olive oil

- Lemon juice
- Oregano and cumin for seasoning
- Garlic, minced

Prep Time: 20 minutes

Cooking Time: 15 minutes

Serving Time: Immediate

Nutritional Info: High in protein, vitamins, and antioxidants

Instructions:

- Marinate chicken cubes with olive oil, lemon juice, minced garlic, oregano, cumin, salt, and pepper.
- Thread chicken, cherry tomatoes, olives, and red onion onto skewers.
- Grill until chicken is cooked through.
- Serve with a side of quinoa or a Greek salad.

Serving Methods:

1. Serve with a dollop of tzatziki sauce for added flavor.
2. Wrap in a whole-grain pita for a delicious sandwich.

Lemon Garlic Grilled Turkey Burgers

Ingredients:

- Ground turkey
- Lemon zest and juice

- Garlic, minced
- Fresh parsley, chopped
- Olive oil
- Salt and pepper to taste

Prep Time: 15 minutes

Cooking Time: 15 minutes

Serving Time: Immediate

Nutritional Info: High in protein, vitamins, and antioxidants

Instructions:

- Mix ground turkey with lemon zest, lemon juice, minced garlic, chopped parsley, olive oil, salt, and pepper.
- Shape into patties and grill until fully cooked.
- Serve with a side of sweet potato wedges or a quinoa salad.

Serving Methods:

1. Top with sliced avocado and tomato for extra freshness.
2. Wrap in lettuce leaves for a low-carb option.

Baked Herb-Crusted Chicken Breast

Ingredients:

- Chicken breasts
- Whole wheat breadcrumbs

- Fresh thyme and rosemary, chopped
- Parmesan cheese, grated
- Dijon mustard
- Garlic, minced
- Olive oil

Prep Time: 15 minutes

Cooking Time: 25 minutes

Serving Time: Immediate

Nutritional Info: High in protein, vitamins, and minerals

Instructions:

- Mix breadcrumbs, chopped thyme, rosemary, Parmesan cheese, Dijon mustard, minced garlic, and olive oil.
- Coat chicken breasts with the mixture and bake until golden.
- Serve with a side of steamed broccoli or a quinoa pilaf.

Serving Methods:

1. Slice and serve over a bed of mixed greens for a light lunch.
2. Pair with a side of roasted Brussels sprouts for a comforting dinner.

Asian-Inspired Grilled Chicken Skewers

Ingredients:

- Chicken thighs, cubed

- Soy sauce (or tamari for gluten-free)

- Sesame oil

- Ginger, grated

- Garlic, minced

- Green onions, sliced

Prep Time: 20 minutes

Cooking Time: 15 minutes

Serving Time: Immediate

Nutritional Info: High in protein, vitamins, and antioxidants

Instructions:

- Marinate chicken cubes in soy sauce, sesame oil, grated ginger, minced garlic, and sliced green onions.

- Thread onto skewers and grill until chicken is cooked through.

- Serve with a side of brown rice or stir-fried vegetables.

Serving Methods:

1. Drizzle with extra soy sauce and sprinkle sesame seeds for added flavor.

2. Serve with a side of Asian slaw for a refreshing option.

Cumin-Spiced Lamb Chops

Ingredients:

- Lamb chops
- Cumin powder
- Coriander powder
- Olive oil
- Lemon juice
- Garlic, minced
- Fresh mint, chopped

Prep Time: 15 minutes

Cooking Time: 15 minutes

Serving Time: Immediate

Nutritional Info: High in protein, vitamins, and healthy fats

Instructions:

- Rub lamb chops with cumin powder, coriander powder, olive oil, lemon juice, minced garlic, and chopped mint.
- Grill until lamb chops are cooked to desired doneness.
- Serve with a side of quinoa or a Greek salad.

Serving Methods:

1. Top with a dollop of tzatziki sauce for extra Mediterranean flavor.
2. Pair with a side of roasted vegetables for a well-balanced meal.

Honey Garlic Glazed Chicken Thighs

Ingredients:

- Chicken thighs, bone-in and skin-on
- Honey
- Soy sauce (or tamari for gluten-free)
- Garlic, minced
- Olive oil
- Dijon mustard

Prep Time: 15 minutes

Cooking Time: 40 minutes

Serving Time: Immediate

Nutritional Info: High in protein, vitamins, and antioxidants

Instructions:

- Mix honey, soy sauce, minced garlic, olive oil, and Dijon mustard to make the glaze.
- Coat chicken thighs with the glaze and bake until golden.
- Serve with a side of roasted sweet potatoes or steamed broccoli.

Serving Methods:

1. Shred leftover chicken and use it in wraps or sandwiches.
2. Pair with a side of quinoa for a filling dinner.

Teriyaki Salmon Steaks

Ingredients:

- Salmon steaks
- Teriyaki sauce (low-sodium)
- Sesame oil
- Ginger, grated
- Garlic, minced
- Green onions, sliced
- Prep Time: 15 minutes

Cooking Time: 15 minutes

Serving Time: Immediate

Nutritional Info: High in omega-3 fatty acids, vitamins, and antioxidants

Instructions:

- Marinate salmon steaks in teriyaki sauce, sesame oil, grated ginger, minced garlic, and sliced green onions.
- Grill until salmon is cooked to desired doneness.
- Serve with a side of brown rice or steamed asparagus.

Serving Methods:

1. Drizzle with extra teriyaki sauce for added flavor.
2. Serve over a bed of sautéed spinach for a light and nutritious meal.

Baked Herb-Marinated Turkey Wings

Ingredients:

- Turkey wings
- Fresh sage and thyme, chopped
- Olive oil
- Lemon juice
- Garlic, minced
- Paprika

Prep Time: 15 minutes

Cooking Time: 1 hour

Serving Time: Immediate

Nutritional Info: High in protein, vitamins, and antioxidants

Instructions:

- Mix chopped sage, thyme, olive oil, lemon juice, minced garlic, and paprika to make the marinade.
- Coat turkey wings with the marinade and bake until golden and cooked through.
- Serve with a side of roasted vegetables or a quinoa salad.

Serving Methods:

1. Shred leftover turkey and use it in salads or wraps.
2. Pair with a side of steamed green beans for a wholesome meal.

Lemon Herb Grilled Chicken Drumsticks

Ingredients:

- Chicken drumsticks
- Lemon zest and juice
- Fresh thyme, chopped
- Garlic, minced
- Olive oil
- Salt and pepper to taste

Prep Time: 15 minutes

Cooking Time: 30 minutes

Serving Time: Immediate

Nutritional Info: High in protein, vitamins, and antioxidants

Instructions:

- Marinate chicken drumsticks in lemon zest, lemon juice, chopped thyme, minced garlic, olive oil, salt, and pepper.
- Grill until chicken is cooked through.
- Serve with a side of quinoa or a green salad.

Serving Methods:

1. Shred leftover chicken and use it in wraps or salads.
2. Serve with a side of roasted sweet potatoes for a filling dinner.

Mango Chili Lime Chicken Skewers

Ingredients:

- Chicken breast, cubed
- Mango, diced
- Chili powder
- Lime juice
- Olive oil
- Cilantro, chopped
- Garlic, minced

Prep Time: 20 minutes

Cooking Time: 15 minutes

Serving Time: Immediate

Nutritional Info: High in protein, vitamins, and antioxidants

Instructions:

- Marinate chicken cubes in diced mango, chili powder, lime juice, chopped cilantro, minced garlic, and olive oil.
- Thread onto skewers and grill until chicken is cooked through.
- Serve with a side of quinoa or a cucumber salad.

Serving Methods:

1. Drizzle with extra lime juice for a burst of freshness.

2. Serve over a bed of brown rice for a more substantial meal.

Spiced Yogurt Marinated Lamb Kebabs

Ingredients:

- Lamb cubes
- Greek yogurt
- Cumin, coriander, and paprika
- Garlic, minced
- Lemon juice
- Olive oil

Prep Time: 20 minutes

Cooking Time: 15 minutes

Serving Time: Immediate

Nutritional Info: High in protein, vitamins, and healthy fats

Instructions:

- Mix Greek yogurt, cumin, coriander, paprika, minced garlic, lemon juice, and olive oil to make the marinade.
- Coat lamb cubes with the marinade and thread onto skewers.
- Grill until lamb is cooked to desired doneness.
- Serve with a side of whole-grain couscous or a green salad.

Serving Methods:

1. Top with a dollop of tzatziki sauce for extra creaminess.

2. Serve with a side of roasted vegetables for a well-balanced meal.

CHAPTER NINE
SEAFOOD RECIPES

Lemon Herb Baked Cod

Ingredients:

- Cod fillets
- Lemon zest and juice
- Fresh dill, chopped
- Garlic, minced
- Olive oil
- Salt and pepper to taste

Prep Time: 15 minutes

Cooking Time: 20 minutes

Serving Time: Immediate

Nutritional Info: High in omega-3 fatty acids, vitamins, and antioxidants

Instructions:

- Mix lemon zest, lemon juice, chopped dill, minced garlic, olive oil, salt, and pepper.
- Coat cod fillets with the mixture and bake until fish is opaque.
- Serve with a side of steamed asparagus or quinoa.

Serving Methods:

1. Top with a spoonful of Greek yogurt for extra creaminess.
2. Serve over a bed of sautéed spinach for a light meal.

Coconut Curry Shrimp

Ingredients:

- Shrimp, peeled and deveined
- Coconut milk
- Curry powder
- Ginger, grated
- Garlic, minced
- Onion, diced
- Olive oil

Prep Time: 20 minutes

Cooking Time: 15 minutes

Serving Time: Immediate

Nutritional Info: High in protein, vitamins, and healthy fats

Instructions:

- Sauté onions, garlic, and ginger in olive oil until softened.
- Add curry powder and coconut milk, then bring to a simmer.
- Add shrimp and cook until pink and opaque.

- Serve over brown rice or cauliflower rice.

Serving Methods:

1. Garnish with chopped cilantro for freshness.
2. Serve with a side of quinoa for added protein.

Grilled Lemon Garlic Salmon

Ingredients:

- Salmon fillets
- Lemon juice and zest
- Garlic, minced
- Fresh parsley, chopped
- Olive oil
- Salt and pepper to taste

Prep Time: 15 minutes

Cooking Time: 15 minutes

Serving Time: Immediate

Nutritional Info: High in omega-3 fatty acids, vitamins, and antioxidants

Instructions:

- Mix lemon juice, lemon zest, minced garlic, chopped parsley, olive oil, salt, and pepper.

- Coat salmon fillets with the mixture and grill until fish is cooked through.
- Serve with a side of roasted Brussels sprouts or quinoa.

Serving Methods:

1. Top with a squeeze of fresh lemon juice for brightness.
2. Serve over a bed of mixed greens for a light lunch.

Miso Glazed Cod

Ingredients:

- Cod fillets
- Miso paste
- Soy sauce (or tamari for gluten-free)
- Mirin
- Green onions, sliced
- Sesame seeds
- Olive oil

Prep Time: 15 minutes

Cooking Time: 20 minutes

Serving Time: Immediate

Nutritional Info: High in protein, vitamins, and antioxidants

Instructions:

- Mix miso paste, soy sauce, mirin, and sliced green onions to make the glaze.
- Coat cod fillets with the glaze and bake until fish is opaque.
- Sprinkle with sesame seeds before serving.
- Serve with a side of steamed broccoli or brown rice.

Serving Methods:

1. Drizzle with extra miso glaze for added flavor.
2. Serve over a bed of quinoa for a more substantial meal.

Garlic Herb Grilled Shrimp Skewers

Ingredients:

- Shrimp, peeled and deveined
- Garlic, minced
- Fresh thyme and rosemary, chopped
- Olive oil
- Lemon juice
- Salt and pepper to taste

Prep Time: 15 minutes

Cooking Time: 5 minutes

Serving Time: Immediate

Nutritional Info: High in protein, vitamins, and antioxidants

Instructions:

- Mix minced garlic, chopped thyme, chopped rosemary, olive oil, lemon juice, salt, and pepper.
- Thread shrimp onto skewers and grill until shrimp are pink and opaque.
- Serve with a side of quinoa or a cucumber salad.

Serving Methods:

1. Dip in a homemade tzatziki sauce for extra flavor.
2. Serve over a bed of mixed greens for a light and refreshing option.

Lemon Dill Baked Halibut

Ingredients:

- Halibut fillets
- Lemon juice and zest
- Fresh dill, chopped
- Garlic, minced
- Olive oil
- Salt and pepper to taste

Prep Time: 15 minutes

Cooking Time: 20 minutes

Serving Time: Immediate

Nutritional Info: High in protein, vitamins, and antioxidants

Instructions:

- Mix lemon juice, lemon zest, chopped dill, minced garlic, olive oil, salt, and pepper.
- Coat halibut fillets with the mixture and bake until fish is opaque.
- Serve with a side of sautéed kale or quinoa.

Serving Methods:

1. Top with a drizzle of extra virgin olive oil for richness.
2. Serve over a bed of wild rice for a heartier meal.

Sesame Ginger Tuna Steaks

Ingredients:

- Tuna steaks
- Soy sauce (or tamari for gluten-free)
- Sesame oil
- Ginger, grated
- Garlic, minced
- Green onions, sliced
- Sesame seeds

Prep Time: 15 minutes

Cooking Time: 10 minutes

Serving Time: Immediate

Nutritional Info: High in protein, vitamins, and healthy fats

Instructions:

- Mix soy sauce, sesame oil, grated ginger, minced garlic, sliced green onions, and sesame seeds.
- Marinate tuna steaks in the mixture and grill until seared on the outside.
- Serve with a side of cauliflower rice or a seaweed salad.

Serving Methods:

1. Garnish with additional sesame seeds for texture.
2. Serve over a bed of zucchini noodles for a low-carb option.

Citrus Marinated Grilled Swordfish

Ingredients:

- Swordfish steaks
- Orange juice and zest
- Lime juice
- Cilantro, chopped
- Olive oil
- Garlic, minced
- Paprika

Prep Time: 15 minutes

Cooking Time: 15 minutes

Serving Time: Immediate

Nutritional Info: High in protein, vitamins, and antioxidants

Instructions:

- Mix orange juice, lime juice, orange zest, chopped cilantro, olive oil, minced garlic, and paprika.
- Marinate swordfish steaks in the mixture and grill until fish is cooked through.
- Serve with a side of roasted sweet potatoes or quinoa.

Serving Methods:

1. Top with a squeeze of fresh lime juice for extra citrus flavor.
2. Serve over a bed of sautéed spinach for a light and nutritious meal.

Cajun Spiced Catfish

Ingredients:

- Catfish fillets
- Cajun seasoning
- Lemon juice
- Olive oil
- Garlic, minced
- Fresh thyme, chopped
- Paprika

Prep Time: 15 minutes

Cooking Time: 15 minutes

Serving Time: Immediate

Nutritional Info: High in protein, vitamins, and antioxidants

Instructions:

- Rub catfish fillets with Cajun seasoning, lemon juice, minced garlic, chopped thyme, and paprika.
- Sauté in olive oil until fish is cooked through.
- Serve with a side of brown rice or a mixed green salad.

Serving Methods:

1. Drizzle with a spicy remoulade sauce for added kick.
2. Serve over a bed of quinoa for a more substantial meal.

Garlic Butter Baked Scallops

Ingredients:

- Scallops
- Butter, melted
- Garlic, minced
- Fresh parsley, chopped
- Lemon juice
- Paprika
- Salt and pepper to taste

Prep Time: 15 minutes

Cooking Time: 15 minutes

Serving Time: Immediate

Nutritional Info: High in protein, vitamins, and healthy fats

Instructions:

- Mix melted butter, minced garlic, chopped parsley, lemon juice, paprika, salt, and pepper.
- Coat scallops with the mixture and bake until scallops are opaque.
- Serve with a side of quinoa or a spinach salad.

Serving Methods:

1. Garnish with additional chopped parsley for freshness.
2. Serve over a bed of cauliflower mash for a low-carb option.

Spicy Thai Basil Shrimp Stir-Fry

Ingredients:

- Shrimp, peeled and deveined
- Thai basil leaves
- Bell peppers, sliced
- Garlic, minced
- Soy sauce (or tamari for gluten-free)

- Sriracha sauce
- Olive oil

Prep Time: 20 minutes

Cooking Time: 10 minutes

Serving Time: Immediate

Nutritional Info: High in protein, vitamins, and antioxidants

Instructions:

- Sauté bell peppers and minced garlic in olive oil until softened.
- Add shrimp and cook until pink and opaque.
- Stir in soy sauce and Sriracha, then toss with Thai basil leaves.
- Serve over brown rice or quinoa.

Serving Methods:

1. Top with crushed peanuts for added crunch.
2. Serve over spiralized zucchini noodles for a low-carb option.

Lemon Garlic Butter Grilled Lobster Tails

Ingredients:

- Lobster tails
- Butter, melted

- Lemon juice and zest
- Garlic, minced
- Fresh chives, chopped
- Paprika
- Salt and pepper to taste

Prep Time: 15 minutes

Cooking Time: 10 minutes

Serving Time: Immediate

Nutritional Info: High in protein, vitamins, and healthy fats

Instructions:

- Mix melted butter, lemon juice, lemon zest, minced garlic, chopped chives, paprika, salt, and pepper.
- Brush lobster tails with the mixture and grill until lobster is cooked through.
- Serve with a side of roasted vegetables or a quinoa salad.

Serving Methods:

1. Garnish with additional chopped chives for freshness.
2. Serve over a bed of wild rice for a more substantial meal.

Cilantro Lime Grilled Mahi-Mahi Tacos

Ingredients:

- Mahi-Mahi fillets
- Cilantro, chopped
- Lime juice and zest
- Garlic, minced
- Cumin and paprika
- Greek yogurt
- Corn tortillas

Prep Time: 20 minutes

Cooking Time: 10 minutes

Serving Time: Immediate

Nutritional Info: High in protein, vitamins, and antioxidants

Instructions:

- Mix chopped cilantro, lime juice, lime zest, minced garlic, cumin, and paprika.
- Marinate Mahi-Mahi fillets in the mixture and grill until fish is cooked through.
- Serve in corn tortillas with a dollop of Greek yogurt.
- Garnish with additional cilantro and lime wedges.

Serving Methods:

1. Top with shredded red cabbage for added crunch.
2. Serve over a bed of shredded lettuce for a lighter option.

Tuscan Style Grilled Swordfish

Ingredients:

- Swordfish steaks
- Sun-dried tomatoes, chopped
- Kalamata olives, sliced
- Fresh basil, chopped
- Garlic, minced
- Balsamic vinegar
- Olive oil

Prep Time: 15 minutes

Cooking Time: 15 minutes

Serving Time: Immediate

Nutritional Info: High in protein, vitamins, and healthy fats

Instructions:

- Mix chopped sun-dried tomatoes, sliced Kalamata olives, chopped basil, minced garlic, balsamic vinegar, and olive oil.
- Marinate swordfish steaks in the mixture and grill until fish is cooked through.
- Serve with a side of roasted sweet potatoes or quinoa.

Serving Methods:

1. Drizzle with extra balsamic vinegar for added richness.

2. Serve over a bed of sautéed spinach for a light and nutritious meal.

Chimichurri Grilled Shrimp Skewers

Ingredients:

- Shrimp, peeled and deveined
- Fresh parsley, chopped
- Cilantro, chopped
- Garlic, minced
- Red wine vinegar
- Olive oil
- Red pepper flakes
- Salt and pepper to taste

Prep Time: 20 minutes

Cooking Time: 5 minutes

Serving Time: Immediate

Nutritional Info: High in protein, vitamins, and antioxidants

Instructions:

- Mix chopped parsley, chopped cilantro, minced garlic, red wine vinegar, olive oil, red pepper flakes, salt, and pepper.
- Thread shrimp onto skewers and grill until shrimp are pink and opaque.

- Serve with a side of brown rice or a mixed green salad.

Serving Methods:

1. Drizzle with extra chimichurri sauce for added flavor.
2. Serve over a bed of quinoa for a more substantial meal.

Salmon and Avocado Sushi Bowls

Ingredients:

- Salmon fillets, cooked and flaked
- Sushi rice, cooked
- Avocado, sliced
- Cucumber, julienned
- Nori strips
- Soy sauce (or tamari for gluten-free)
- Pickled ginger

Prep Time: 30 minutes

Cooking Time: 15 minutes

Serving Time: Immediate

Nutritional Info: High in omega-3 fatty acids, vitamins, and antioxidants

Instructions:

- Arrange sushi rice in bowls and top with flaked salmon, sliced avocado, julienned cucumber, and nori strips.

- Serve with soy sauce and pickled ginger on the side.
- Garnish with sesame seeds and chopped green onions.

Serving Methods:

1. Drizzle with a spicy mayo sauce for added kick.
2. Serve over a bed of mixed greens for a lighter option.

Shrimp and Broccoli Stir-Fry

Ingredients:

- Shrimp, peeled and deveined
- Broccoli florets
- Soy sauce (or tamari for gluten-free)
- Sesame oil
- Ginger, grated
- Garlic, minced
- Brown rice

Prep Time: 20 minutes

Cooking Time: 10 minutes

Serving Time: Immediate

Nutritional Info: High in protein, vitamins, and antioxidants

Instructions:

- Sauté broccoli florets in sesame oil until slightly tender.

- Add shrimp, grated ginger, and minced garlic, and stir-fry until shrimp are pink and opaque.
- Stir in soy sauce and serve over brown rice.

Serving Methods:

1. Top with sliced green onions for freshness.
2. Serve over cauliflower rice for a low-carb option.

Crispy Baked Coconut Shrimp

Ingredients:

- Shrimp, peeled and deveined
- Coconut flakes
- Whole wheat breadcrumbs
- Egg whites
- Lime juice
- Paprika
- Olive oil

Prep Time: 20 minutes

Cooking Time: 15 minutes

Serving Time: Immediate

Nutritional Info: High in protein, vitamins, and healthy fats

Instructions:

- Dip shrimp in egg whites, then coat with a mixture of coconut flakes, whole wheat breadcrumbs, lime juice, and paprika.
- Bake until shrimp are golden and crispy.
- Serve with a side of mango salsa or a quinoa salad.

Serving Methods:

1. Dip in a homemade pineapple dipping sauce for extra flavor.
2. Serve over a bed of mixed greens for a light and refreshing option.

Lemon Pepper Grilled Tuna Steaks

Ingredients:

- Tuna steaks
- Lemon zest and juice
- Black pepper
- Olive oil
- Garlic, minced
- Fresh thyme, chopped

Prep Time: 15 minutes

Cooking Time: 10 minutes

Serving Time: Immediate

Nutritional Info: High in protein, vitamins, and antioxidants

Instructions:

- Mix lemon zest, lemon juice, black pepper, olive oil, minced garlic, and chopped thyme.
- Marinate tuna steaks in the mixture and grill until seared on the outside.
- Serve with a side of quinoa or a cucumber salad.

Serving Methods:

1. Drizzle with extra virgin olive oil for added richness.
2. Serve over a bed of brown rice for a more substantial meal.

Mediterranean Style Baked Red Snapper

Ingredients:

- Red snapper fillets
- Cherry tomatoes, halved
- Kalamata olives, sliced
- Red onion, thinly sliced
- Olive oil
- Lemon juice
- Fresh oregano, chopped
- Garlic, minced

Prep Time: 20 minutes

Cooking Time: 20 minutes

Serving Time: Immediate

Nutritional Info: High in omega-3 fatty acids, vitamins, and antioxidants

Instructions:

- Mix halved cherry tomatoes, sliced Kalamata olives, thinly sliced red onion, olive oil, lemon juice, chopped oregano, and minced garlic.
- Place red snapper fillets on a baking sheet and top with the Mediterranean mixture.
- Bake until fish is cooked through.
- Serve with a side of couscous or a Greek salad.

Serving Methods:

1. Garnish with additional chopped oregano for freshness.
2. Serve over a bed of quinoa for a more substantial meal

CHAPTER TEN
MEAL PLAN

Day 1:

Breakfast: Lemon Garlic Grilled Turkey Burgers with Avocado

Lunch: Coconut Curry Shrimp with Cauliflower Rice

Dinner: Baked Herb-Crusted Chicken Breast with Quinoa Pilaf

Day 2:

Breakfast: Asian-Inspired Grilled Chicken Skewers with Brown Rice

Lunch: Lemon Herb Baked Cod with Steamed Asparagus

Dinner: Spicy Thai Basil Shrimp Stir-Fry with Brown Rice

Day 3:

Breakfast: Cumin-Spiced Lamb Chops with Greek Yogurt

Lunch: Miso Glazed Cod with Roasted Brussels Sprouts

Dinner: Lemon Dill Baked Halibut with Sautéed Kale

Day 4:

Breakfast: Honey Garlic Glazed Chicken Thighs with Quinoa

Lunch: Chimichurri Grilled Shrimp Skewers with Mixed Greens

Dinner: Tuscan Style Grilled Swordfish with Roasted Sweet Potatoes

Day 5:

Breakfast: Teriyaki Salmon Steaks with Brown Rice

Lunch: Cajun Spiced Catfish with Brown Rice

Dinner: Garlic Herb Grilled Shrimp Skewers with Quinoa Salad

Day 6:

Breakfast: Lemon Pepper Grilled Tuna Steaks with Cucumber Salad

Lunch: Crispy Baked Coconut Shrimp with Mango Salsa

Dinner: Salmon and Avocado Sushi Bowls

Day 7:

Breakfast: Mediterranean Style Baked Red Snapper with Greek Salad

Lunch: Tuscan Style Grilled Swordfish with Quinoa

Dinner: Spiced Yogurt Marinated Lamb Kebabs with Roasted Vegetables

Day 8:

Breakfast: Lemon Garlic Grilled Turkey Burgers with Avocado

Lunch: Coconut Curry Shrimp with Cauliflower Rice

Dinner: Baked Herb-Crusted Chicken Breast with Quinoa Pilaf

Day 9:

Breakfast: Asian-Inspired Grilled Chicken Skewers with Brown Rice

Lunch: Lemon Herb Baked Cod with Steamed Asparagus

Dinner: Spicy Thai Basil Shrimp Stir-Fry with Brown Rice

Day 10:

Breakfast: Cumin-Spiced Lamb Chops with Greek Yogurt

Lunch: Miso Glazed Cod with Roasted Brussels Sprouts

Dinner: Lemon Dill Baked Halibut with Sautéed Kale

Day 11:

Breakfast: Honey Garlic Glazed Chicken Thighs with Quinoa

Lunch: Chimichurri Grilled Shrimp Skewers with Mixed Greens

Dinner: Tuscan Style Grilled Swordfish with Roasted Sweet Potatoes

Day 12:

Breakfast: Teriyaki Salmon Steaks with Brown Rice

Lunch: Cajun Spiced Catfish with Brown Rice

Dinner: Garlic Herb Grilled Shrimp Skewers with Quinoa Sala

Day 13:

Breakfast: Lemon Pepper Grilled Tuna Steaks with Cucumber Salad

Lunch: Crispy Baked Coconut Shrimp with Mango Salsa

Dinner: Salmon and Avocado Sushi Bowls

Day 14:

Breakfast: Mediterranean Style Baked Red Snapper with Greek Salad

Lunch: Tuscan Style Grilled Swordfish with Quinoa

Dinner: Spiced Yogurt Marinated Lamb Kebabs with Roasted Vegetables

Day 15:

Breakfast: Lemon Garlic Grilled Turkey Burgers with Avocado

Lunch: Coconut Curry Shrimp with Cauliflower Rice

Dinner: Baked Herb-Crusted Chicken Breast with Quinoa Pilaf

Day 16:

Breakfast: Asian-Inspired Grilled Chicken Skewers with Brown Rice

Lunch: Lemon Herb Baked Cod with Steamed Asparagus

Dinner: Spicy Thai Basil Shrimp Stir-Fry with Brown Rice

Day 17:

Breakfast: Cumin-Spiced Lamb Chops with Greek Yogurt

Lunch: Miso Glazed Cod with Roasted Brussels Sprouts

Dinner: Lemon Dill Baked Halibut with Sautéed Kale

Day 18:

Breakfast: Honey Garlic Glazed Chicken Thighs with Quinoa

Lunch: Chimichurri Grilled Shrimp Skewers with Mixed Greens

Dinner: Tuscan Style Grilled Swordfish with Roasted Sweet Potatoes

Day 19:

Breakfast: Teriyaki Salmon Steaks with Brown Rice

Lunch: Cajun Spiced Catfish with Brown Rice

Dinner: Garlic Herb Grilled Shrimp Skewers with Quinoa Salad

Day 20:

Breakfast: Lemon Pepper Grilled Tuna Steaks with Cucumber Salad

Lunch: Crispy Baked Coconut Shrimp with Mango Salsa

Dinner: Salmon and Avocado Sushi Bowls

Day 21:

Breakfast: Mediterranean Style Baked Red Snapper with Greek Salad

Lunch: Tuscan Style Grilled Swordfish with Quinoa

Dinner: Spiced Yogurt Marinated Lamb Kebabs with Roasted Vegetables

CHAPTER ELEVEN

STAYING ACTIVE AND HEALTHY

Exercise Recommendations for Seniors

Exercise is crucial for maintaining overall health and well-being, especially for seniors. Regular physical activity can help improve cardiovascular health, maintain muscle mass and strength, enhance flexibility, and contribute to a better quality of life. However, it's important for seniors to engage in exercises that are safe and suitable for their individual needs and health conditions.

Here are some exercise recommendations for seniors:

Aerobic Exercise:

- ***Walking:*** A low-impact exercise that can be easily adapted to individual fitness levels.
- Swimming or Water Aerobics: Gentle on the joints and provides resistance for muscle strengthening.
- ***Cycling:*** Stationary or outdoor cycling can improve cardiovascular health without putting excessive stress on the joints.

Strength Training:

- ***Bodyweight Exercises:*** Squats, lunges, and wall push-ups can help maintain muscle strength.

- **_Resistance Band Exercises:_** These provide resistance for muscle building without the need for heavy weights.
- **_Light Weights:_** Incorporate light dumbbells for upper body strength training, ensuring proper form and control.

Flexibility and Stretching:

- **_Yoga:_** Promotes flexibility, balance, and relaxation.
- **_Tai Chi:_** A gentle Chinese martial art that enhances balance, flexibility, and overall mobility.
- **_Daily Stretching Routine:_** Focus on major muscle groups to maintain flexibility and prevent stiffness.

Balance Exercises:

- **_Single Leg Stands:_** Holding onto a stable surface, lift one leg at a time to improve balance.
- **_Heel-to-Toe Walk:_** Walk in a straight line placing the heel of one foot directly in front of the toes of the other.
- **_Balance Exercises on an Unstable Surface:_** Use balance pads or cushions to challenge stability.

Cardiovascular Exercise:

- **_Elliptical Trainer:_** Provides a low-impact, full-body workout.
- **_Recumbent Biking:_** Offers cardiovascular benefits with added back support.
- **_Low-Impact Aerobics:_** Follow exercise routines designed for seniors to improve heart health.

Adapted and Specialized Programs:

- *Silver Sneakers:* A fitness program designed for older adults, often offered through Medicare plans.
- *Senior Fitness Classes:* Participate in classes tailored to seniors, including dance, aerobics, or senior yoga.

Regular Physical Activity:

- *Daily Walks:* Aim for at least 30 minutes of brisk walking most days of the week.
- *Gardening:* Engage in light gardening activities to stay active.
- *Household Chores:* Activities like vacuuming, sweeping, and light cleaning contribute to physical activity.

Consultation with Healthcare Professionals:

Before starting any exercise program, seniors should consult with their healthcare provider to ensure the chosen activities are safe and suitable for their health conditions.

If there are pre-existing health concerns, a physical therapist or certified fitness professional with experience in senior fitness can provide personalized guidance.

Stress Management and Relaxation Techniques

Stress management and relaxation techniques play a pivotal role in maintaining overall well-being, especially in today's fast-paced and demanding world. Chronic stress can contribute to a range of physical and mental health issues, making it essential for individuals to incorporate effective stress-reducing strategies into their daily lives. Here, we will professionally discuss various stress management and relaxation techniques:

1. Stress Management Techniques:

Mindfulness Meditation:

- Mindfulness involves focusing on the present moment without judgment. Meditation techniques, such as mindful breathing or body scan, can help individuals become more aware of their thoughts and emotions, reducing stress.

Progressive Muscle Relaxation (PMR):

- PMR involves systematically tensing and then relaxing different muscle groups. This technique helps release physical tension and promotes a sense of calm.

Cognitive Behavioral Therapy (CBT):

- CBT is a therapeutic approach that helps individuals identify and change negative thought patterns contributing to stress. It equips individuals with coping strategies to manage stressors effectively.

Time Management:

- Efficiently organizing and prioritizing tasks can alleviate the feeling of being overwhelmed. Creating a realistic schedule and setting achievable goals can contribute to a sense of control.

Physical Activity:

- Regular exercise is a powerful stress reducer. Physical activity releases endorphins, which act as natural mood lifters, and provides an opportunity to clear the mind.

Journaling:

- Writing down thoughts and feelings can be a cathartic process. Journaling allows individuals to gain insights into stress triggers and explore positive perspectives.

Social Support:

- Maintaining strong social connections provides emotional support during challenging times. Sharing concerns with friends, family, or support groups can help reduce the burden of stress.

2. Relaxation Techniques:

Deep Breathing Exercises:

- Diaphragmatic or abdominal breathing helps activate the body's relaxation response. Inhale deeply through the nose, allowing the abdomen to expand, and exhale slowly through pursed lips.

Guided Imagery:

- Visualization of calming scenes or positive experiences can promote relaxation. Guided imagery exercises involve creating detailed mental images to evoke a sense of peace.

Aromatherapy:

- Inhaling pleasant scents, such as lavender or chamomile, can have a calming effect. Aromatherapy can be incorporated through essential oils, candles, or diffusers.

Progressive Relaxation Techniques:

- Similar to PMR, progressive relaxation involves systematically tensing and relaxing muscle groups, promoting a sense of physical and mental calmness.

Yoga and Tai Chi:

- These mind-body practices combine physical postures, controlled breathing, and meditation. They help improve flexibility, balance, and overall relaxation.

Music and Art Therapy:

- Engaging in activities like listening to soothing music or creating art can provide an outlet for self-expression and relaxation.

Hot Baths or Showers:

- Warm water can help relax muscles and soothe the nervous system. Adding calming scents like lavender to bathwater can enhance the experience.

3. Professional Guidance:

Therapeutic Counseling:

- Seeking the support of a licensed therapist or counselor can provide an opportunity to explore and address stressors in a structured and confidential setting.

Biofeedback:

- Biofeedback techniques involve monitoring physiological responses to stress, such as heart rate and muscle tension, and learning how to control these responses for relaxation.

Mind-Body Programs:

- Participating in structured programs that integrate mindfulness, meditation, and relaxation techniques, such as Mindfulness-Based Stress Reduction (MBSR), can be beneficial.

CONCLUSION

In conclusion, the exploration of the "Blood Type A Diet for Seniors" has provided a comprehensive understanding of tailored nutrition for individuals with blood type A, focusing on its potential benefits for senior health. The overview highlighted the specific characteristics of blood type A individual, emphasizing the importance of personalized dietary choices.

Tailoring the diet to blood type A involves selecting foods that support optimal digestion, nutrient absorption, and immune function. Understanding the unique characteristics of blood type, A individual, such as their potential susceptibility to stress and the benefits of incorporating calming activities, allows for a more holistic approach to senior well-being.

The discourse on the blood type A diet showcased the significance of including a variety of nutrient-rich foods, aligning with the blood type A recommendation. The inclusion of specific recipes for breakfast, lunch, dinner, snacks, and desserts further demonstrated the diversity and flexibility of the diet, providing seniors with a range of delicious and nutritious options.

The 21-day meal plan offers a practical implementation of the blood type A diet, incorporating a variety of recipes to ensure a balanced and enjoyable eating experience. It takes into account the nutritional needs of seniors, promoting not only physical health but also considering the importance of mental and emotional well-being.

Ultimately, the blood type A diet for seniors is a personalized and holistic approach to nutrition, taking into account individual differences and preferences. While the information and meal plan provided serve as a valuable guide, it's crucial for individuals to consult with healthcare professionals or nutritionists to tailor the recommendations based on their specific health profiles, ensuring a safe and effective dietary approach for senior well-being.